Anti-Inflammatory Cookbook for Beginners

Unlock Your Well-Being with 2000 Days of Delicious, Home-Cooked Recipes to Boost Immunity and Conquer Inflammation. Includes 12-Week Meal Plan

By

Nathan Terrell

Contents

Introduction

Inflammation is seen as a threat to health by many people. But inflammation is actually a defense mechanism your body uses on its own. Inflammation is typically the end result of a cascade of chemical events triggered by hormones in the body as it attempts to rid itself of pathogens or restore chemical equilibrium. There is clearly something wrong when our bodies react with inflammation and agony. This may result from a dietary shortage, an over buildup of nutrients, or an attack by microorganisms. Inflammation in the body has been linked to numerous diseases and disorders, including diabetes, cancer, heart disease, COPD, and Alzheimer's.

On the other side, many elements have been shown to help lessen and even cure inflammation. Reducing stress, keeping a regular exercise routine, and watching what you eat are all good places to start. The food we eat greatly affects the way our bodies function. This is because the foods we eat shape our bodies, and avoiding those that promote inflammation can greatly improve our overall health.

Some diets have been shown to reduce inflammation and other illness symptoms. Anti-inflammatory diets are defined as those that aim to minimize inflammation. These diets consist of carefully chosen foods that provide nutrients while also offering soothing compounds that aid in reducing inflammation.

That's the whole point of the book! Therefore, this book is exactly what you need to improve your health and lessen inflammation. In addition, a 30-day meal plan is included, as well as advice on how to eat healthier with diet, lifestyle changes and physical activity.

Changing your diet and way of life is made easier with the help of this book. The more information you have, the closer you reach your goal. Good luck!

Part 1: Introduction

Overview of Inflammation and Its Impact on Health

Inflammation is a normal process in the body that happens in response to injury, infection, or discomfort. It is an essential component of the immune system's defense process, aiding in the healing of injured tissues and the battle against harmful microorganisms. However, when inflammation becomes chronic or protracted, it can have serious consequences for one's health.

Chronic inflammation has been related to various health problems, including heart disease, diabetes, obesity, autoimmune disorders, and some cancers. It's also linked to symptoms like pain, weariness, edema, and joint stiffness. Furthermore, persistent inflammation can hasten the aging process and hasten the development of age-related disorders.

Chronic inflammation is frequently caused by unhealthy lifestyle behaviors such as a poor diet, a sedentary lifestyle, stress, insufficient sleep, and exposure to environmental contaminants. These variables can cause an overactive immune response, resulting in chronic inflammation throughout the body.

Understanding the effects of inflammation on health is essential for living an anti-inflammatory lifestyle. Individuals can help prevent and decrease the negative effects of chronic inflammation by making intentional decisions to reduce inflammation, such as eating a nutrient-rich diet, engaging in regular physical activity, controlling stress levels, prioritizing sleep, and avoiding dangerous substances.

Reduced inflammation not only increases overall well-being but it also plays an important role in disease prevention and longevity. Individuals can improve their health, increase their energy levels, improve their mental clarity, maintain a healthy weight, and lower their risk of chronic diseases by adopting an anti-inflammatory lifestyle.

While an anti-inflammatory lifestyle can benefit most people, it is always best to seek personalized advice and guidance from healthcare professionals or registered dietitians, especially if you have specific health conditions or dietary restrictions.

Individuals can improve their well-being, vitality, and longevity by recognizing the influence of inflammation on health and adopting an anti-inflammatory lifestyle.

Chapter 1: What is Inflammation?

What images or thoughts come to mind when you consider inflammation? Inflammation is the root cause of almost all modern diseases, manifesting externally as redness, swelling, heat, and pain but also beginning within. It's vital to understand what happens inside your body when inflammation is present before we delve into discussing how you may change your diet to help combat systemic inflammation. You can do a lot to protect your body from inflammatory disorders if you have a firm grasp on what inflammation is and what causes inflammation.

When your body detects an invader, such as bacteria or a virus, it triggers inflammation, which uses white blood cells and also the substances they make to defend against infection.

In diseases like arthritis, however, the immune system induces inflammation regardless of whether there are no outside invaders present. Autoimmune diseases occur when the body's immune system incorrectly harms healthy tissues, believing them to be contaminated or aberrant.

The first step is realizing that not all inflammation is harmful. In truth, inflammation aids in recovery and serves as a defense mechanism against illness and infection.

1.1 Acute and Chronic Inflammation

There are two different kinds of inflammation: acute and chronic.

1.1.1 Acute Inflammation

Inflammation can either be short-term (acute) or long-term (chronic). The immune system's response to foreign invaders is acute inflammation. It's only temporary. The presence of dangerous microorganisms or tissue injury is the most common trigger of acute inflammation. In most cases, acute inflammation does not require emergency care and can be treated easily. CBD oil (to reduce inflammation), compression, and rest are all effective treatments. Acute inflammation can be helpful to a person's health, but its aftereffects need to be addressed to prevent further injury or infection, both of which can result in excruciating pain. For instance, a broken bone can worsen if not properly cared for.

Acute inflammation is relatively mild and simple to treat. Since the symptoms are so blatant, a diagnosis can be made quickly.

Signs of Acute Inflammation

The following are the main signs of acute inflammations:

- Redness
- Lack of function
- Swelling
- Heat
- Pain

1.1.2 Chronic Inflammation

Slow, persistent inflammation that lasts for months or even years is known as chronic inflammation. The initial injury and the body's capacity for recovery play a role in how severe chronic inflammation becomes.

This type of inflammation has far-reaching and persistent impacts on the body. Due to its persistent character, low-grade inflammation is sometimes known by this name. The list of ailments it can trigger is surprisingly long. Inflammation at a low level suggests an immunological response to internal dangers. Chronic inflammation may also induce illnesses like stroke and heart attack, although the consequences on your system and the process involved are little understood at present.

Signs of Chronic Inflammation

The following are the main signs of chronic inflammations:

- Joint pain
- Digestive problems
- Swelling of joints and feeling warm

- Fatigue
- Energy loss
- Skin issues (acne, eczema, psoriasis)
- Fever
- Headaches
- Mood disorders (anxiety, depression)
- Redness
- Trouble sleeping
- Muscle fitness
- Joint stiffness
- Trouble losing weight
- Chills

Chronic Inflammation Causes

Chronic inflammation is caused by various factors, including injury or infection, excessive exposure to irritants (polluted air or chemicals), and an autoimmune condition (the immune system mistakenly attacks healthy cells and tissues).

These causes, however, do not affect everyone because every human body responds differently to things. There are also cases of chronic inflammation with no discernible etiology. Chronic inflammation, according to specialists, is enabled by a variety of conditions such as chronic stress, obesity, smoking, alcohol, and many more.

How Chronic Inflammation Affects the Body

When the body's inflammatory reaction is persistent, healthy organs, tissues, and cells might be harmed. If this persists for an extended period of time, it can result in internal scarring, death of tissues, and DNA damage. All of this might contribute to a decline in an individual's overall health.

Internal scarring, DNA damage, and tissue death all share one feature. They all contribute to the development of numerous diseases in the body, including type 2 diabetes, heart disease, cancer, asthma, rheumatoid arthritis, obesity, and neurological diseases such as Alzheimer's disease.

1.2 Health Effects of Chronic Inflammation

Chronic inflammation can be fatal; according to estimates, 3 out of every 5 people die from inflammatory illnesses. Inflammation poses numerous health concerns, the most serious of which are listed here.

1.2.1 Rheumatoid Arthritis (RA):

Let's just say that inflammation makes arthritis almost unbearable. A person's movements are hampered, and it occasionally hurts while talking and eating. The patient's permanent tissue damage may occur from a chronic state of swelling in the joints. Patients with arthritis are therefore advised to keep this inflammation under control and to explore new ways to do so.

1.2.2 Psoriasis

Another immune-mediated disease in which the patient may experience large patches of inflammation on the skin. It causes skin redness and irritation and typically appears on the elbows, scalp, and knees. If the problem is not dealt with promptly, the swelling may worsen.

1.2.3 Asthma

Asthma is a respiratory disorder in which the human respiratory system's internal lining swells, constricts the air pathways, and causes shortness of breath. Chronic asthma can even be fatal for the patients. To treat this disease, immediate anti-inflammatory measures are essential, but patients are also advised to avoid taking any substances that could provoke this reaction.

1.2.4 Inflammatory Bowel Disease (IBD)

Inflammation occurs inside the digestive tract and swells the internal lining of the intestines in this disorder, also known as Crohn's disease. It causes gut pain, fatigue, diarrhea, and sometimes weightlessness. Controlling inflammation can help prevent severe pain and suffering in this disease.

1.2.5 Diabetes

Inflammation can result in insulin resistance, prediabetes, and, eventually, diabetes. Pancreatic inflammation can damage insulin-producing beta cells, eventually leading to diabetes. Diabetes patients should be extra cautious of cell or tissue damage because their bodies may not respond adequately to the injuries.

1.2.6 Obesity

Obesity and inflammation are inextricably related. Cronin inflammation may lead to alleviating the rate of metabolism and unnecessary fat deposition. Fat cells may contribute to further inflammation, and thus the cycle continues. Obesity and inflammation should be addressed before they become critical.

1.2.7 Heart Disease

Any blockage in blood flow affects the functioning of the cardiac muscles. Inflammation frequently constricts blood vessels, resulting in increased internal pressure. It then affects the heart, which might result in temporary or permanent damage.

1.3 Why Is It Important to Reduce Inflammation?

It's critical to reduce chronic inflammation in your body because it's not supposed to be there! Your body cannot function properly in the midst of inflammation. You can alleviate inflammatory-caused symptoms such as those described above by lowering inflammation.

Above all, when you're inflammation-free, you feel your best. When you are at your best, you live purposefully, and your cup is brimming with opportunities to serve others. And this has a knock-on effect.

Chapter 2: Basics of the Anti-Inflammatory Diet

Anti-inflammatory diets have been in the limelight for quite some time as a terrific diet to improve our general health. There is a lot of evidence that these diets lower inflammation in the body, which lowers our risks of getting sick, whether it's the average cold or a more serious illness. While an anti-inflammatory diet can benefit anyone's health, it is especially beneficial for those of us who suffer from inflammatory disorders such as arthritis, gout, lupus, and scleroderma since it helps to minimize the systemic inflammation that comes with these conditions.

You are what you eat, as the saying goes. If you put processed, inflammation-causing foods into your body, you will produce inflammation, which can result in undesired reactions such as digestive pain, skin issues, mood changes, and even disease. If you fuel your body with potent inflammation-fighting foods that are high in phytonutrients and have the ability to combat disease, you are giving your body what it needs to perform at its best. An anti-inflammatory diet focuses on exactly that, providing your body with the nutrients it requires to thrive.

The anti-inflammatory diet consists of entire, unprocessed foods. These healthful foods work to naturally lower inflammation in your body, thereby preventing disease.

When consuming anti-inflammatory foods, there are still many delectable items that may be consumed and incorporated into your daily diet. Eliminating foods that are refined, processed, high in sugar, grain-fed animal products, alcohol, or contain excessive caffeine will significantly aid in lessening general inflammation in your body.

2.1 Key Concepts of the Anti-Inflammatory Diet

The anti-inflammatory diet focuses on eating foods that have been found to lower inflammation and increase general health. Here are several key anti-inflammatory diet concepts:

2.1.1 Focus on Whole and Unprocessed Foods

Fruits, vegetables, legumes, whole grains, and lean proteins should be prioritized. These meals are high in nutrients and antioxidants, which aid in the fight against inflammation.

2.1.2 Include Omega-3 Fatty Acids

Include omega-3 fatty acid sources such as fatty fish (salmon, sardines, mackerel), chia seeds, flaxseeds, and walnuts in your diet. Omega-3 fatty acids have anti-inflammatory effects.

2.1.3 Opt for Healthy Fats

Select healthy fats such as olive oil, avocados, and almonds. These fats have anti-inflammatory properties and promote overall heart health.

2.1.4 Include Anti-Inflammatory Spices and Herbs

Use herbs and spices such as turmeric, ginger, cinnamon, garlic, and rosemary. These spices are anti-inflammatory powerhouses.

2.1.5 Include Colorful Vegetables and Fruits

Consume a wide range of colorful fruits and vegetables, as they include phytonutrients and antioxidants that help to reduce inflammation.

2.1.6 Reduce your Intake of Processed Foods

Reduce your intake of processed and refined foods, such as processed meats, sugary snacks, and packaged meals. These foods are frequently high in chemicals and trans fats, both of which can lead to inflammation.

2.1.7 Increase Antioxidant Intake

Choose berries, tomatoes, dark leafy greens, and green tea high in antioxidants. Antioxidants shield the body from oxidative damage and inflammation.

2.1.8 Gluten and Dairy Intolerance

If you have gluten or dairy sensitivities or intolerances, consider decreasing or eliminating these foods. In some people, these can contribute to inflammation.

2.1.9 Limit your Intake of Added Sugars

Limit your intake of added sugars, which might contribute to inflammation. Choose natural sweeteners such as honey or healthier alternatives such as stevia or monk fruit extract.

2.1.10 Stay Hydrated

Drink plenty of water during the day to stay hydrated. Water aids in the removal of pollutants and improves general bodily functions.

2.1.11 Practice Mindful Eating

Pay attention to hunger and fullness cues to practice mindful eating. Eat carefully and savor your meals to completely appreciate the flavors and textures of the cuisine.

2.1.12 Lifestyle Factors

In addition to eating a nutritious diet, reengage in regular physical activity, manage stress, get enough sleep, and avoid smoking and excessive alcohol intake. These lifestyle factors can also help to reduce inflammation.

2.2 Benefits of an Anti-Inflammatory Diet

Many people who follow this diet wish to minimize inflammation throughout their bodies in order to prevent or reduce the amount of pain they experience, particularly in their joints. However, there are some other health benefits that you may be able to obtain by following this diet plan, and some of them may even surprise you; we will look at the key ones.

2.2.1 Lowers Chronic Inflammation

Chronic inflammation has been linked to various health problems, including heart disease, obesity, diabetes, and certain types of cancer. An anti-inflammatory diet promotes better overall health and lowers the risk of chronic diseases by lowering inflammation in the body.

2.2.2 Heart Health Improvements

A heart-healthy diet is high in anti-inflammatory foods such as fruits, vegetables, whole grains, and healthy fats. This diet can help lower blood pressure, LDL cholesterol levels, and the risk of heart disease and stroke.

2.2.3 Improve Cellular Health

Chronic inflammation can affect insulin signaling and compromise cellular function, leading to insulin resistance. An anti-inflammatory diet promotes optimal cellular health and increases the body's ability to manage blood sugar levels by consuming nutrient-dense meals and lowering inflammation.

2.2.4 Diabetes Prevention

Adopting an anti-inflammatory diet can also aid in diabetes prevention. Insulin resistance and the emergence of type 2 diabetes are both connected to chronic inflammation. You can enhance insulin sensitivity and lessen your chance of getting diabetes by lowering inflammation with an anti-inflammatory diet.

2.2.5 Weight Control

The capacity to boost your overall metabolism is the most significant advantage of following an anti-inflammatory diet. Metabolism, or the pace at which your body burns calories, has a direct impact on how quickly you lose weight. You will lose weight faster if you have a high metabolism. It will be far more difficult to lose those excess pounds if you have a slow metabolism.

2.2.6 Immune Function Enhancement

The anti-inflammatory diet emphasizes foods that are high in antioxidants, vitamins, and minerals. These nutrients promote a healthy immune system, enhancing the body's ability to fight infections and disorders.

2.2.7 Better Digestion
The anti-inflammatory diet is high in fiber, which is one of the key components that helps your body digest food efficiently. Beneficial bacteria in your stomach aid in the digestion and absorption of certain vitamins and minerals, and their absence can result in health problems such as constipation. You may enhance digestion and reduce the probability of digestive disorders by increasing your fiber intake and ensuring that the beneficial bacteria are healthy.

2.2.8 Improved Cognitive Function
Chronic inflammation has been linked to memory loss and neurodegenerative disorders such as Alzheimer's. An anti-inflammatory diet high in brain-healthy nutrients, including omega-3 fatty acids, antioxidants, and vitamins, can improve cognitive performance and protect against age-related decline.

2.2.9 Balanced Blood Sugar Levels
An anti-inflammatory diet helps regulate blood sugar levels by focusing on whole foods and limiting processed sugars, lowering the risk of type 2 diabetes, insulin resistance, and metabolic syndrome.

2.2.10 Reduces Bloating
A low-inflammatory diet can help reduce bloating and digestive pain. Many inflammatory meals, including processed foods, refined sugars, and artificial chemicals, can cause bloating and digestive irritation. You may maintain a healthy gut and prevent bloating by replacing these items with complete, nutrient-dense options.

2.2.11 Skin Health Improvements
Inflammation is linked to several skin diseases, including acne, eczema, and psoriasis. By lowering inflammation and encouraging a healthy complexion, an anti-inflammatory diet can help improve skin health.

2.2.12 Increased Vitality and Energy
Nutrient-dense foods supply the body with critical vitamins, minerals, and antioxidants, which help with energy levels, mood, and general vitality.

Chapter 3: Inflammatory Foods to Avoid

3.1 Foods with Anti-Inflammatory Properties

Avoid foods that may induce or increase inflammation to regulate and minimize inflammation. The anti-inflammatory diet also includes a list of foods to avoid. Among these foods are the following.

3.1.1 Foods High in Fructose and Sugar

Sugary foods and foods containing a lot of fructose are at the top of our list of foods to avoid. In our daily diet, two main causes lead to inflammation. The first is high fructose corn syrup, whereas the second is table sugar. These are the two most common forms of sugar in our modern diet. According to one study, these additional sugars cause significant harm to the body.

A high-sucrose diet may increase your risk of developing breast cancer, claims another study. Sucrose is a kind of sugar. Additionally, there is evidence to support the idea that consuming sugary meals can impede or obstruct the anti-inflammatory benefits of omega-3 fatty acids.

Fructose and the other sugars found naturally in all of our foods are not inherently nasty or evil. They're actually beneficial because they provide the body with the energy it requires. What's dangerous is taking in too much, which may happen quickly.

Simply drinking a large can of Coke will provide your body with all of the sugar it requires in one week in one session. Do you, however, stop at one can of soda? Some folks consume three or more drinks every day.

Chronic illnesses such as cancer, obesity, diabetes, insulin resistance, fatty liver disease, and chronic kidney disease have been related to high fructose intake.

Foods with high levels of added sugar include the following:

- Cookies
- Certain types of cereals
- Fruit juices (sweetened ones)
- Sweet pastries
- Chocolates
- Doughnuts
- Cakes
- Soft drinks
- Any sugar-sweetened drinks
- Candy

3.1.2 Processed Cooking Oil

Most common cooking oils have been depleted of all nutrients. They also have a high omega-6 fatty acid content and a low omega-3 fatty acid content. This imbalance causes inflammation, which contributes to both heart disease and cancer.

Avoid the following oils:

- Grape seed oil,
- safflower oil,
- corn oil,
- cottonseed oil
- sunflower oil

Look for these oils on the ingredient lists of processed foods and fast food restaurants.

3.1.3 Alcoholic Drinks
The acidity of alcohol induces inflammation of the esophagus and larynx. Furthermore, the yeast found in alcohol irritates the stomach and digestive tract linings. Continued alcohol consumption causes liver damage. Repeated alcohol abuse causes chronic inflammation, which can lead to certain illnesses and malignancies.

Avoid the following:

- Liquor
- beer
- Wine

3.1.4 Processed Meat
Beef jerky, smoked meat, bacon, ham, and sausages are examples of processed meat. They're delicious, and some individuals have made them dinner table standards. However, research indicates that these meals are linked to an increased risk of several ailments, including colon cancer, diabetes, stomach cancer, and heart disease.

Colon cancer is the most common disease linked to processed meat eating. Researchers believe this is because these meats contain a high concentration of advanced glycation end products or AGEs. When meat is combined with other ingredients and then heated to high temperatures, AGEs occur.

AGEs trigger inflammation in the body, according to research. It is important to note that several variables contribute to the development of colon cancer. However, research indicates that the most significant contributing factor is most likely the consumption of processed meat and the associated inflammation.

Beef, pork, and any smoked meats should be avoided.

3.1.5 Refined Grains, Breads, and Pastries
According to research, high carbohydrate consumption increases the risk of inflammation. Breads and pastries significantly increase carbohydrate levels. Because processed grains lack fiber and vitamin B, they are essentially nutritionally deficient and insulin-stimulating. Furthermore, they contain gluten, a component that irritates the gut lining and causes inflammation.

Avoid the following:

- white rice
- boxed cereals
- pasta
- white bread
- biscuits
- pastries, and noodles

3.1.6 Refined Carbohydrates
Carbohydrates, as the principal source of glucose, are plainly not advised for the majority of people. Carbohydrates, on the other hand, have the potential to influence inflammation as well as blood sugar and insulin levels. Because refined carbohydrates have a higher (GI) glycemic index than the rest of the carbs, they are the most harmful. One study found that older persons who eat a lot of high-GI foods have a 2.9 greater risk of dying from an inflammatory disease (Buyken et al., 2010). The clearest example is chronic

obstructive pulmonary disease (COPD). White bread can boost blood sugar levels and the amount of a certain inflammatory marker on its own. Cookies, cakes, chocolates, some cereals, pastries, pasta, bread, sugary soft drinks, and any processed item having extra flour or sugar have refined carbs.

3.1.7 Trans Fats
The fight against trans fats continues. It contributes to the world's bad diet. Trans fats raise bad cholesterol while decreasing good cholesterol. Cholesterol levels can trigger inflammation on a very deep coronary level. This can result in heart problems and cancer.

Avoid the following:

- deep-fried food
- commercial baked items
- fast food

Remember: If a food label states 0 g trans-fat, it may not be accurate if you live in the United States. The United States government permits trans-fat concentrations of 0.5 g or less to be labeled as 0 g trans-fat on packaging. Avoid processed foods at all costs.

3.7 Gluten Grains

Gluten is present in all breads and pastries. Gluten is a protein that causes digestive difficulties in many people. It also causes back and joint pain, irritable bowel syndrome, and skin problems. Gluten intolerance is becoming more common. It is advisable to avoid indigestible protein entirely.

Avoid the following:

- barley
- cereal
- rye
- candy
- kamut
- pasta

3.1.8 Gluten Grains

Gluten is present in all breads and pastries. Gluten is a protein that causes digestive difficulties in many people. It also causes back and joint pain, irritable bowel syndrome, and skin problems. Gluten intolerance is becoming more common. It is advisable to avoid indigestible protein entirely.

Avoid the following:

- barley
- cereal
- rye
- candy
- kamut
- pasta

3.1.9 Dairy Products

In the years after infancy, over 60% of the human population cannot digest the major component of dairy, lactose. Lactose can cause inflammation in the form of stomach pain, diarrhea, acne, constipation, and breathing difficulties. Lactose should be avoided.

Avoid the following:

- Butter
- Cheese
- Milk
- Cottage cheese
- Cream cheese
- Frozen yogurt
- Ice cream
- cream sauces
- Milk and cream

3.1.10 Corn
Corn is a food to avoid because so much of it is genetically modified these days. In the United States, over 90% of corn is genetically altered. Genetically modified organisms (GMOs) or genetically modified foods are new to our food system and can offer major health risks. They can inhibit the immune system and cause inflammation as a result of the changes. Corn is common in processed meals; for example, high-fructose corn syrup is included in the vast majority of processed, sugary desserts. Furthermore, vegetable oils like corn oil have more omega-6 fatty acids, which are similarly inflammatory.

Avoid this corn-containing foods to avoid:

- Corn
- Corn oil
- High-fructose
- Corn flour
- Corn starch
- Dextrin
- Corn sugar
- Corn tortillas
- Dextrose
- Golden syrup
- Corn syrup
- Xanthan gum
- Maltodextrin
- Maize
- Cornmeal
- Maltose

3.1.11 Caffeine
Can't live without your morning caffeine fix or an afternoon pick-me-up? If you have inflammation, you should consider quitting caffeine. Caffeine causes the stomach to release its contents early, allowing undigested food to enter the small intestine and irritate the digestive tract. Caffeine elevates blood pressure and pulse rate, suppresses appetite, and interferes with sleep. Caffeine also strains the neurological system, which can interfere with cortisol levels, the final nail in the caffeine coffin. Because cocoa (and any chocolate product) contains caffeine, some practitioners advise avoiding raw cocoa powder as well.

3.1.12 Soy
Like corn, this contentious bean is a common allergen. According to a recent assessment from the US Department of Agriculture's Economic Research Service, 93 percent of soy farmed in the United States is genetically modified. Soy has a lot of goitrogens, which are chemicals that decrease thyroid activity. Soy also contains anti-nutrients, including phytates and oxalates, which interfere with digestion and affect the endocrine system.

Avoid this soy food:

- Bean curd
- Tempeh
- Miso
- Soybeans
- Edamame
- Soy flakes

- Soy ice cream
- Soy milk
- Soy isolate
- Soy lecithin
- Soy nut butter
- Tofu
- Soy nuts
- Soy oil
- Soy protein
- Soy sauce
- Soy yogurt
- Tamari
- Soy flour

3.2 Suggestions for Eliminating These Foods from the Diet

3.2.1 Opt for Unprocessed Foods
Choose items that have not been processed. These foods are nutrition dense and low in inflammatory compounds.

3.2.2 Check the Labels!
Read the labels on packaged foods thoroughly before purchasing. Sugary, fatty, and chemically-enhanced items should be avoided.

3.2.3 In-House Cooking
Use fresh ingredients to cook delicious meals at home. This gives you more say over what goes into your food and how it's prepared, giving you more control over your inflammation intake.

3.2.4 Eat More Foods High in Antioxidants
Eat lots of berries, nuts, leafy greens, and seeds to get the antioxidant protection you need. In addition to reducing inflammation, antioxidants also protect cells from harm.

3.2.5 Replace Unhealthy Fats
Olive oil, avocado oil, and coconut oil are all excellent alternatives to vegetable oil full of omega-6 fatty acids.

3.2.6 Cut Back on Processed Meats
Reduce your intake of processed meats like bacon, sausage, and deli meats because they typically have unhealthy additives and excessive sodium. Choose unprocessed meats like lean meats and plant-based proteins.

3.2.7 Reduce Added Sugars
Reduce your intake of sugary foods and drinks. If you want something sweet, try honey or some fresh fruit instead of refined sugar.

3.2.8 Mindful Cooking
Instead of frying, which might promote the development of hazardous chemicals, try grilling, steaming, baking, or sautéing.

3.2.9 Maintain a Healthy Fluid Balance
To cut down on your consumption of added sugars and artificial sweeteners, try switching to water, herbal teas, or unsweetened beverages instead of sugary drinks.

3.2.10 Think Ahead

Prepare your meals and snacks ahead of time so you don't have to get anything quick. Make a few nutritious meals and snacks on Sunday to keep on hand all week.

Chapter 4: Anti-Inflammatory Foods to Include

4.1 List of Foods with Anti-Inflammatory Properties

Inflammation is your body's method of alerting you that something is wrong, which, as you've discovered, isn't always easy to determine. It won't always be obvious, like the discomfort in your joints from arthritis, but it will be something you generally dismiss or are unaware of. Food cravings, moodiness, persistent weariness, and digestive issues are all symptoms of inflammation.

The most crucial factor to consider is whether the diet is acidic or alkaline. The pH of the body is described using the phrases alkaline and acidity. When you eat mostly alkaline foods, your body will be alkaline as well. When you eat mostly acidic foods, your body becomes acidic, causing inflammation. An alkaline body makes a person feel active and free of joint pain and allows the body to function properly. Your body will naturally desire healthy, fresh meals in order to maintain its overall health. You won't feel well all the time if you have an acidic body, and you'll be sluggish. A couple of unhealthy habits might lead to a slew of other health issues. Inflammation can be accelerated by a lack of sleep, junk food, smoking, and alcohol consumption.

Your lifestyle and dietary choices are your two most powerful anti-inflammatory defenses. Here are some foods that help to fight inflammation to get you started on the right track.

4.1.1 Natural Sweeteners

Because artificial sweeteners and refined sugars harm the digestive system, natural sweeteners can deliver a wonderful flavor boost.

Look for: Brown rice syrup, coconut syrup, stevia, and honey.

4.1.2 Gluten-Free Grains

When gluten is removed from the equation, grains become incredibly nutritious. Quinoa, for example, is a superfood packed with protein, fiber, iron, and manganese. These grains provide numerous benefits without damaging the stomach lining or causing joint and back pain.

Look for: Buckwheat, whole rice, teff, quinoa, and millet.

4.1.3 Cold-pressed, Unrefined Oils

To meet your oil needs, look for unrefined oils in jars. These oils do not promote inflammation; they are also associated with healthy fats and sufficient nutrition.

Look for: Avocado oil, mustard seed oil, olive oil, coconut oil, and sesame seed oil.

4.1.4 Substitute for Milk

In the aftermath of "no dairy," look to dairy replacements to meet all of your milk demands. Dairy alternatives are frequently fortified with healthy proteins and pleasant flavors, and they pose no dietary constraints.

Look for: Almond milk, brown rice milk, rice milk, and hemp seed milk are all options.

4.1.5 Legumes and Beans

Beans and legumes are high in protein as well as proper carbs. They are high in fiber, which promotes healthy digestion.

Look for: Kidney beans, chickpeas, and adzuki.

4.1.6 Meat

Limit your red meat consumption to once or twice a week (or avoid it entirely if possible), and choose organic, free-range chicken, turkey, eco-friendly fish, lamb, and wild game.

4.1.7 Fresh Vegetables

Vegetables account for almost half of the inflammatory diet. These vegetables provide a wealth of vitamins, minerals, and phytonutrients to the body. Furthermore, these components work together to provide proper fuel to the body's cells. As a result, the body may operate and recover at a consistent rate without becoming bogged down in the inflammatory process for too long. Furthermore, the fiber in vegetables facilitates digestion without the stumbling blocks associated with an inflamed digestive tract.

Look for: Bright peppers, celery, spinach, broccoli, kale, and zucchini.

4.1.8 Dark Leafy Greens
Dark leafy greens contain antioxidant vitamins A, C, E, and K, which fight cellular damage and inflammation. They're also high in anti-inflammatory omega-3 fatty acids and B vitamins, which help with stress management and nervous system nourishment.

4.1.9 Allium Vegetables
Onions, garlic, leeks, ramps, shallots, scallions, and chives all have several health benefits. Onions are high in vitamin C and quercetin, which aids in the relief of allergy symptoms. Garlic is no slouch either; it has antiviral and antibacterial qualities as well as a variety of sulfurous components that reduce inflammation throughout the body.

4.1.10 Root Vegetables
Anti-inflammatory and antioxidant powerhouses include carrots, sweet potatoes, rutabaga, parsnips, celery root, turnips, and beets. Carrots and sweet potatoes are high in vitamin A, which serves to nourish the mucosal cells in the digestive tract, improve vision, strengthen the immune system, and keep skin healthy. Sweet potatoes have anthocyanin pigments, while beets contain betalains, both of which inhibit the development of inflammatory enzymes.

4.1.11 Basil
Eugenol, a volatile oil discovered in basil, inhibits the enzymes that cause inflammation (the same enzymes that NSAIDs target).

4.1.12 Berries
Blueberries, blackberries, raspberries, and strawberries are high in antioxidants, which fight cellular damage and block enzymes that cause inflammation. Berries are also abundant in fiber, which is good for your digestion, cardiovascular system, and blood sugar levels.

4.1.13 Dill
This herb aids in the neutralization of carcinogens and is used to treat digestive issues such as gas, indigestion, and constipation.

4.1.14 Fennel
This delicious vegetable inhibits the mechanisms that cause inflammation. Antioxidants and immune-boosting elements are also found in fennel.

4.1.15 Fish
Omega-3 fatty acids—the good fats—are abundant in wild salmon, sardines, mackerel, anchovies, and halibut. Salmon, in particular, is high in two omega-3 fatty acids known as EPA and DHA, which aid in producing anti-inflammatory molecules.

4.1.16 Pineapple
Bromelain, found in the core and stem of this tropical fruit, lowers inflammation and aids protein digestion.

4.1.17 Ginger
Gingerols, anti-inflammatory chemicals found in its root, inhibit pro-inflammatory molecules. Ginger is used to cure a wide range of ailments, including digestive problems, nausea, colds, motion sickness, headaches, arthritis, and flu.

4.1.18 Turmeric
Curcumin is responsible for turmeric's anti-inflammatory properties. It can aid in the reduction of inflammation caused by inflammatory bowel disease, cystic fibrosis, arthritis, and cancer.

4.1.19 Avocados
Avocados are high in monounsaturated fats, magnesium, fiber, and potassium, all of which are beneficial to the heart. Because they contain tocopherols and carotenoids, their nutritional content reduces cancer risk.

4.1.20 Green Tea
This is the healthiest beverage since it lowers the risk of heart disease, obesity, and Alzheimer's disease. This is because they have anti-inflammatory and antioxidant properties.

4.1.21 Peppers
Peppers and chilies are high in vitamin C and antioxidants, both of which have anti-inflammatory properties. The product's sinapic and ferulic acids prevent inflammation and aging.

4.1.22 Cherries
They are high in antioxidants such as catechins and anthocyanin, which help to prevent inflammation.

4.1.23 Grapes
They contain anthocyanin, which helps to alleviate inflammation. It also lowers the risk of developing diseases such as diabetes, obesity, heart disease, eye condition, and Alzheimer's disease. Grapes also contain resveratrol, which lowers blood pressure, protects the brain, relieves joint pain, promotes insulin sensitivity, and suppresses cancer cells.

4.1.24 Dark Chocolate
In a study on the effects of cocoa on lab mice, researchers discovered that the antioxidant component of cocoa helped to lower the mice's blood sugar levels and stopped them from gaining weight. They also discovered that gut bacteria convert chocolate into anti-inflammatory and heart-healthy chemicals that inhibit genes that promote inflammation and insulin resistance. Eat some chocolate with apple slices for excellent outcomes. The apple will accelerate the fermentation process in the gut, resulting in weight loss and inflammation reduction. Make certain that you consume the proper type of chocolate. The optimal cacao content is 70% or more.

4.1.25 Tomatoes
Tomatoes are also nightshade, but they can help some people reduce inflammation. Lycopene levels are high in red, juicy tomatoes. Lycopene has been shown to help reduce inflammation in the body and lungs. It also specifically helps with the inflammation that causes depression. Lycopene is found in the skin of tomatoes, so tossing a handful of cherry tomatoes into a salad is an excellent method to absorb the antioxidant. Cooking tomatoes enhances the lycopene content.

4.1.26 Nuts and Certain Seeds
Nuts and seeds include high levels of both beneficial fats and protein. These healthy fats curb hunger, keeping one's mind off of manufactured foods. Furthermore, they are high in omega-3 fatty acids, aiding appropriate brain cell transmission.

Look for: Almonds, Brazil nuts, macadamia nuts, flax seeds, pumpkin seeds, chia seeds, hemp seeds, and walnuts.

4.2 How These Foods Help Reduce Inflammation in the Body
These foods are packed with certain elements that help reduce the inflammation in our bodies. Here's the list of elements present in these foods which help get rid of inflammation.

4.2.1 Antioxidants
Antioxidant-rich foods, such as berries, leafy greens, and dark chocolate, aid in the neutralization of free radicals in the body. Free radicals are highly reactive chemicals that can cause oxidative damage and inflammation. Antioxidants aid in the protection of cells and the reduction of inflammation.

4.2.2 Fatty Acids Omega-3
Fatty fish, such as salmon and sardines, are abundant in omega-3 fatty acids, which have anti-inflammatory qualities. Omega-3 fatty acids aid in the reduction of inflammatory chemicals such as cytokines and prostaglandins in the body.

4.2.3 Phytonutrients
Many plant-based foods, such as ginger, turmeric, and tomatoes, contain anti-inflammatory phytonutrients. Curcumin in turmeric and gingerol in ginger, for example, have been found to block inflammatory pathways in the body.

4.2.4 Monounsaturated Fats

Olive oil, which is high in monounsaturated fats, contains a molecule called oleocanthal, which has been shown to have anti-inflammatory properties similar to NSAIDs. Monounsaturated fats aid in lowering the body's synthesis of inflammatory markers.

4.2.5 Fiber

Fiber-rich foods, such as leafy greens and almonds, promote a healthy gut microbiome. A healthy gut microbiome is linked to less inflammation and better immune function.

4.2.6 Flavonoids

Flavonoids, which have anti-inflammatory qualities, are found in green tea and dark chocolate. Flavonoids aid in decreasing inflammation by inhibiting particular enzymes involved in the inflammatory response.

4.2.7 Lycopene

Tomatoes are high in lycopene, an antioxidant that has been demonstrated to reduce inflammatory markers. Lycopene may also lower the risk of chronic inflammatory disorders such as heart disease and some malignancies.

You may assist in reducing inflammation and boosting overall health by integrating these items into your diet. It is critical to remember that a well-balanced and diverse diet, as well as a healthy lifestyle, are essential for efficiently managing inflammation.

Chapter 5: Meal Planning in the Anti-Inflammatory Diet

The foundation of the anti-inflammatory diet is the preparation of well-balanced, nourishing meals. You may get the most out of the anti-inflammatory effects of the foods you eat by selecting and using them with purpose. In addition to reducing stress and freeing up time during the week, the benefits of weekly meal preparation are numerous.

The following are some tips to keep in mind when planning meals on the anti-inflammatory diet:

5.1 Practical Tips for Planning Balanced, Anti-Inflammatory Meals

5.1.1 Be Sure to Use a Rainbow of Colorful Produce

Eat a rainbow of fruits and veggies, and aim to fill half your plate with them. They contain anti-inflammatory antioxidants and phytochemicals in abundance. Pick a wide range of colors and varieties to get a wide range of vitamins and minerals.

5.1.2 Whole Grains Should Be Prioritized

Instead of white rice, white flour pasta, and white bread, try whole grains like brown rice, oats, quinoa, and whole wheat bread. Compared to refined grains, whole grains provide more fiber and minerals that help lower inflammation.

5.1.3 Go for Lean Protein

Eat more skinless chicken, fish, and legumes for healthy, low-fat protein. These foods are a good source of the amino acids the body needs to grow and repair itself.

5.1.4 Pick the Good Fats

Avocados, almonds, seeds, olive oil, fatty seafood, and other healthy fat sources should be incorporated into your diet. Omega-3 fatty acids and other anti-inflammatory chemicals are found in these fatty acids.

5.1.5 Add Some Flavor

Herbs and spices are great anti-inflammatory additions to food. Anti-inflammatory qualities can be found in several spices, including turmeric, ginger, cinnamon, garlic, and rosemary.

5.1.6 Cut Down on Processed Foods

Avoid or limit your consumption of processed foods, which frequently contain artificial ingredients, trans fats, and excessive amounts of salt and sugar. These factors may exacerbate existing inflammatory conditions.

5.1.7 DIY Meals

When at all possible, cook meals at home. This puts you in charge of what goes into your food, how it's prepared, and whether or not it has any inflammatory chemicals.

5.1.8 The Importance of Preparation

Put some thought into your weekly food preparations. As a result, you'll be less likely to resort to harmful takeout or convenience foods and more likely to eat a wide range of nutritious, inflammation-fighting foods.

5.1.9 It's Important to Stay Hydrated

Hydrate yourself and maintain good health by drinking lots of water throughout the day. For appropriate biological functions, including the reduction of inflammation, proper hydration is crucial.

5.1.10 Control Your Serving Sizes

Keep your nutrient intake in check by paying attention to your portion sizes. When excess calories are stored as fat, inflammation is exacerbated.

5.2 Tips for Meal Preparation and Time Management

5.2.1 Make a Meal Plan
Plan your meals for the week ahead at the start of each week. This will help you keep track of the supplies and prevent you from running out.

5.2.2 Keep the Recipes Basic
Five to ten major ingredients (not including spices and herbs) are a good range to work with when cooking. Try to find meals that can be put together in 30 minutes or less with little effort from you. Because of the negative effects of pain on enjoyable activities like cooking and gardening, you should reduce meal preparation to a minimum.

Prepare meals easily by employing techniques and aids that reduce stress on your muscles and joints.

5.2.3 Stock Up on Quick-and-Easy Foods
Get some frozen veggies and fruits and some canned beans that are low in salt. These are useful to have on hand as a backup if you go several days without going to the grocery store due to a lack of energy or pain. If you need a quick supper without a lot of cutting, stock up on pre-cut salads, vegetables, and fruit.

5.2.4 Preparing Food in Bulk
Consider doing batch cooking on weekends or in your spare time. Prepare larger amounts of certain meals and store them in single-serving containers. This will save you time during the week and make it easier to get a nutritious dinner when you're pressed for time.

5.2.5 Plan Your Meals Around Your Routine
When you feel less tired and discomfort, make the most of it. It's normal to have weeks where more meals and snacks can be made than others.

5.2.6 Prepare the Ingredients Ahead of Time
Prepare ingredients such as meat and vegetables for marinating or grains in advance. Assembling meals will go more quickly and efficiently.

5.2.7 Used Freezer-Friendly Meals
Meals that can be frozen and used at a later time should be prepared. It's easy to freeze and reheat dishes like casseroles, soups, and stews.

5.2.8 Repurpose the Extras
Don't throw away any extra food. Make use of the day-old chicken by transforming it into a chicken salad, or use the cooked vegetables in a stir-fry.

5.2.9 Keep a Well-Stocked Pantry
Store dry items, canned products, and spices in your kitchen pantry. Having the necessary components on hand for speedy and healthy meal preparation is made much easier with a well-stocked pantry.

5.2.10 Invest in Time-Saving Kitchen Tools
You can save a lot of time by purchasing time-saving kitchen appliances, such as a food blender, processor, or mandolin slicer.

You can modify the meal-planning procedure to fit your tastes and schedule. If you want to keep your meals interesting and fulfilling, try out new recipes, flavors, and combinations. Meal planning can be a useful tool in aiding your anti-inflammatory journey if you use it to make well-considered food selections and put your body's nourishment first.

Chapter 6: Managing Food Intolerances

6.1 What is Food Intolerance?
Some people have trouble digesting, absorbing, or metabolizing the nutrients in specific foods. Unlike food allergies, which are immune system reactions, food intolerances are related more to the digestive system than the immunological system. Food intolerance symptoms might be comparable to food allergy symptoms but are typically milder. Bloating, stomach pain, nausea, headaches, vomiting, and exhaustion are all common signs of food intolerance.

6.2 What are the Roots of Food Intolerance?
Most cases of food intolerance can be traced back to an individual's inability to digest specific food components such as lactose in dairy, gluten in wheat, or histamine in fermented foods. Food additives, including sulfites & monosodium glutamate (MSG), have been linked to food intolerances. Food poisoning, insufficient production of digestive enzymes, and sensitivity to chemicals in food are some possible reasons for food intolerance.

6.3 Common Food Intolerances Related to Inflammation
Food intolerances can cause inflammation in the body and aggravate pre-existing inflammation. Here are some typical food intolerances associated with inflammation:

6.3.1 Gluten Intolerance
Gluten is a protein discovered in grains such as barley, wheat, and rye. Gluten intolerance, also known as non-celiac gluten sensitivity or celiac disease, is characterized by an immunological response to gluten that causes inflammation in the small intestine. This inflammation has the potential to spread to other parts of the body, resulting in a variety of symptoms and problems.

6.3.2 Lactose Intolerance
Lactose is a type of sugar that is found in dairy products. Lack of lactase, an enzyme necessary to digest lactose, is the root cause of lactose intolerance. Lactose consumption can cause digestive symptoms like gas, bloating, and diarrhea. Inflammation in the digestive system can occur as a result of the body's failure to digest lactose effectively.

6.3.3 Sensitivities to Food Additives
Certain food additives, like artificial preservatives, flavors, and colorings, have been shown to cause inflammation in certain people. These additives can be found in packaged snacks, processed foods, and sauces. Inflammation can be reduced by carefully reading food labels and avoiding goods containing known trigger ingredients.

6.3.4 Histamine Intolerance
Histamine is a chemical that has a role in the body's immunological response. Some people have trouble metabolizing histamine, resulting in a buildup of this molecule in the body. Histamine-rich foods, like aged cheeses, fermented meals, and some shellfish, can cause inflammation in those with histamine sensitivity.

6.3.5 FODMAP Intolerance
FODMAPs (fermentable oligosaccharides, disaccharides, monosaccharides, and polyols) are a type of carbohydrate that can cause digestive problems and inflammation in the small intestine. Certain fruits, vegetables, cereals, and sweeteners are examples of high-FODMAP foods. Individuals suffering from IBS or other digestive issues may be susceptible to FODMAPs.

6.4 Tips on How to Identify and Manage Food Intolerances
Food intolerances can be difficult to identify and manage, particularly if you are unsure which foods are responsible for your pain. With a little effort, you may simply determine the items to avoid and enhance your general health.

Here are some pointers to help you figure out which foods you need to avoid and how to manage food intolerances:

6.4.1 Determine your Triggers

Identifying the foods that cause your symptoms is the first step in managing food intolerance. Maintain a food journal in which you document the things you eat as well as the symptoms you feel. This will assist you in identifying patterns and determining which foods are triggering your problems.

6.4.2 Maintain a Food Diary

Begin by keeping a diary of everything you consume and drink, noting the time of day and any side effects. This can assist you in identifying patterns and determining which foods contribute to your discomfort.

6.4.3 Dietary elimination

Try removing one meal or food group from your diet for a while to see if your signs improve. Once you've discovered the offending food, consider eliminating it entirely from your diet.

6.4.4 Replace your Trigger Foods

It can be helpful to locate adequate alternatives while attempting to avoid trigger foods. If you have trouble digesting lactose, for instance, you might want to look into lactose-free milk or other dairy-free options. Try some gluten-free bread or spaghetti if you have a gluten intolerance.

6.4.5 Get Yourself Tested

If you're unsure which foods contribute to your discomfort, talk to your doctor about being examined for food intolerances. Food allergies and intolerances can be identified using blood tests & skin prick tests.

6.4.6 Examine Food Labels

Always carefully check food labels to identify potential intolerances and allergens. Peanuts, dairy, wheat, tree nuts, and soy products are common allergies.

6.4.7 Home Cooking

Home cooking is a good strategy for managing food intolerance. It enables you to manage the ingredients in your meals and guarantee that they are free of trigger foods. Experiment with fresh ingredients and recipes to ensure your meals are both tasty and filling.

6.4.8 Consult with a Registered Dietitian

A licensed dietician can assist you in developing a specific diet plan that meets your dietary requirements while avoiding foods that aggravate your symptoms.

To summarize, identifying which foods to stay away from if you have a food intolerance might be difficult, but it is feasible with the support of a medical professional and some initiative on your part. Keeping a food diary, experimenting with an exclusion diet, getting examined, checking food labels, and obtaining assistance from a trained dietitian are all useful ways to manage food intolerance.

Keep in mind that avoiding offending foods is only one part of managing food intolerance. You can improve your health and well-being by switching to healthier options, eating at home more often, and adopting other healthy habits. If you're willing to put in the time and effort, you can learn to live with your food intolerance.

Part 2: Anti-Inflammatory Recipes

Introduction to the Recipes

Welcome to the nutritious and tasty world of anti-inflammatory dishes! In this section, we've carefully handpicked a range of delectable dishes that are not only pleasing to the palate but also packed with anti-inflammatory components. These recipes are intended to help you on your way to a healthier, inflammation-free life.

In these recipes, anti-inflammatory foods like colorful fruits and vegetables, whole grains, lean meats, healthy fats, and various herbs and spices take center stage. Each dish is carefully designed to give a balance of flavors, textures, and nutrients while minimizing inflammatory triggers.

Recipe Preparation and Ingredient Selection Tips

Choose Fresh and Whole Foods: Fresh, seasonal fruits and vegetables, whole grains, and lean proteins are all good choices. These raw and minimally processed foods are high in nutrients and low in chemicals that can cause inflammation.

Embrace Colorful Produce: Include a wide range of bright fruits and vegetables in your meals. The brilliant colors imply a wide range of anti-inflammatory antioxidants and phytochemicals.

Healthy Fats: Avocados, almonds, seeds, and extra virgin olive oil are all good sources of healthy fats. These fats have anti-inflammatory characteristics and may aid in food absorption.

Make It More Interesting: Experiment with various herbs and spices recognized for their anti-inflammatory properties. Turmeric, ginger, garlic, cinnamon, and cayenne pepper are a few examples of ingredients that can add flavor as well as health benefits to your recipes.

Mindful Cooking Techniques: Instead of deep frying, use methods such as steaming, sautéing, grilling, or baking. These procedures help to preserve the nutritional integrity of the components while reducing the amount of oil used.

Variety and Balance: Aim for a balanced diet by combining macronutrients such as proteins, healthy fats, and complex carbohydrates. Variate your recipe selections to provide various nutrients to help with general health and well-being.

Keep in mind that these recipes are intended to inspire and guide you on your anti-inflammatory journey. Feel free to modify them to suit your tastes and dietary requirements. By adding these dishes to your daily routine, you are taking proactive measures to nourish your body, reduce inflammation, and embrace a healthy lifestyle. One tasty food at a time, enjoy the journey to well-being!

Chapter 7: Breakfast and Snacks

1. Golden Milk Chia Pudding
Preparation time: 10 minutes | **Cooking time:** 0 minutes | **Serves:** 4

Per Serving: Calories 337 | Total Fat 11g | Protein 10g | Carbs 51g | Fiber: 2g

Ingredients:

- ½ teaspoon of ground cinnamon
- 4 cups of coconut milk
- ½ teaspoon of ground ginger
- 3 tablespoons of honey
- 1 teaspoon of ground turmeric
- ¾ cup of coconut yogurt
- 1 cup of fresh mixed berry
- ¼ cup of toasted coconut chips
- ½ cup of chia seeds

Directions:

- Inside a mixing dish, combine the coconut milk, cinnamon, honey, turmeric, and ginger. Incorporate the coconut yogurt.
- Inside a separate bowl, add the berries, chia seeds, and coconut chips.
- Add the milk mixture.
- Set aside for 6 hours in the refrigerator to chill.

2. Savory Breakfast Pancakes
Preparation time: 5 minutes | **Cooking time:** 6 minutes | **Serves:** 4

Per Serving: Calories 108 | Total Fat 2g | Protein 2g | Carbs 20g | Fiber: 0.5g

Ingredients:

- 1 cup of coconut milk
- ½ cup of almond flour
- ¼ teaspoon of ground black pepper
- ½ cup of tapioca flour
- 1 teaspoon of salt
- ½ teaspoon of chili powder
- 1 handful of chopped cilantro leaves
- ¼ teaspoon of turmeric powder
- ½ red onion, chopped
- ½ inch ginger, grated

Directions:

- Into a mixing dish, add all of the ingredients till thoroughly mixed.
- Grease a pan and heat it on low to medium flame.
- 1/4 cup batter should be poured onto the pan and spread to form a pancake.

- Cook for 3 minutes on each side.
- Serve and enjoy.

3. Scrambled Eggs with Smoked Salmon
Preparation time: 10 minutes | **Cooking time:** 10 minutes | **Serves:** 2

Per Serving: Calories 349 | Total Fat 12g | Protein 29g | Carbs 3g | Fiber: 2g

Ingredients:
- 4 slices of chopped wild-caught smoked salmon
- Fresh chives, chopped
- 4 eggs
- 2 tablespoons of coconut milk
- Salt to taste

Directions:
- Inside a mixing bowl, combine the egg, coconut milk, and chives.
- Heat the skillet over a medium-low flame with oil.
- Place the egg batter in the pan and scramble it as it cooks.
- When the eggs begin to settle, add the smoked salmon and simmer for 2 minutes more.
- Serve and enjoy!

4. Breakfast Burgers with Avocado Buns
Preparation time: 10 minutes | **Cooking time:** 5 minutes | **Serves:** 1

Per Serving: Calories 458 | Total Fat 39g | Protein 13g | Carbs 20g | Fiber: 14g

Ingredients:
- 1 lettuce leaf
- 1 ripe avocado
- Sesame seeds for garnishing
- 1 egg, pasture-raised
- 1 tomato slice
- Salt to taste
- 1 red onion slice

Directions:
- Cut the avocado in half. It will work like the bun. Place aside.
- Cook the egg sunny-side up in a skillet over medium flame for 5 minutes or till it's set.
- Assemble the morning burger by layering the egg, onion, tomato, and lettuce leaf on top of one avocado half. Place the remaining avocado bun on top.
- Top with sesame seeds and season using salt.

5. Kiwi Strawberry Smoothie
Preparation time: 10 minutes | **Cooking time:** 0 minutes | **Serves:** 1

Per Serving: Calories 250 | Total Fat 1g | Protein 0.1g | Carbs 34g | Fiber: 4.3g

Ingredients:

- 1 peeled and chopped kiwi
- 1/2 cup of fresh or frozen strawberries, chopped
- 1 cup of almond or coconut milk
- 1 teaspoon of ground basil
- 1 teaspoon of turmeric
- 1 banana, diced
- 1/4 cup of chia seed powder

Directions:

- In a food processor, combine all of the ingredients.
- Drink immediately after thoroughly mixing all of the ingredients.

6. Breakfast Omelet

Preparation time: 10 minutes | **Cooking time:** 10 minutes | **Serves:** 2

Per Serving: Calories 210 | Total Fat 14g | Protein 15g | Carbs 5g | Fiber: 2g

Ingredients:

- 1 red bell pepper, diced
- 1 teaspoon of herb seasoning
- 2 eggs, beaten
- ½ cup of mushrooms, sliced
- 1 stalk of green onion, chopped

Directions:

- In a mixing dish, whisk together the eggs. Stir in the remaining ingredients.
- Fill a small baking pan halfway with the egg mixture. Place the pan inside the oven.
- Cook for 10 minutes at 350°F in the oven.

7. Breakfast Avocado Boat

Preparation time: 10 minutes | **Cooking time:** 10 minutes | **Serves:** 2

Per Serving: Calories 458 | Total Fat 38g | Protein 20g | Carbs 14g | Fiber: 2g

Ingredients:

- 1 bell pepper, chopped
- 2 avocados, sliced in half and pitted
- Pepper to taste
- 2 tomatoes, chopped
- 2 tablespoons of cilantro, chopped
- ¼ onion, chopped
- 4 eggs

Directions:

- Cut the avocado flesh into small pieces. Place in a mixing bowl.
- Except for the eggs, stir in the remaining ingredients.

- Refrigerate for around 30 minutes.
- On top of the avocado shell, crack the egg.
- Preheat your oven at 350°F. Bake for 7 to 8 minutes.
- Put avocado salsa on top.

8. Fruity Flaxseed Breakfast Bowl
Preparation time: 10 minutes | **Cooking time:** 5 minutes | **Serves:** 1

Per Serving: Calories 480 | Total Fat 26g | Protein 39g | Carbs 41g | Fiber: 2g

Ingredients:

For the Porridge:

- 1 medium banana, mashed
- ¼ cup of flaxseeds, freshly ground
- A pinch of fine-grained sea salt
- 1 cup of almond or coconut milk
- ¼ teaspoon of cinnamon, ground

For the Toppings:

- Walnuts, chopped and raw
- Blueberries, fresh or defrosted
- Pure maple syrup (optional)

Directions:

- Combine all of the porridge ingredients in a medium-sized saucepan over medium flame. For 5 minutes, or till the porridge thickens and reaches a low boil, stir regularly.
- In a serving bowl, place the cooked porridge. Garnish with the desired toppings and drizzle with maple syrup if desired.

9. Blueberry Smoothie
Preparation time: 10 minutes | **Cooking time:** 0 minutes | **Serves:** 1

Per Serving: Calories 431 | Total Fat 21g | Protein 10g | Carbs 56g | Fiber: 8g

Ingredients:

- 1 teaspoon of Maca powder
- 1 cup of almond milk
- 2 handfuls of spinach
- 1 cup of frozen blueberries
- ¼ teaspoon of cinnamon
- 1 frozen banana
- ¼ teaspoon of cayenne pepper
- 1 tablespoon of almond butter

Directions:

- In a blender, combine all of the ingredients until well incorporated. Serve right away.

10. Kale Turmeric Scramble
Preparation time: 10 minutes | **Cooking time:** 10 minutes | **Serves:** 1

Per Serving: Calories 137 | Total Fat 8g | Protein 13g | Carbs 8g | Fiber: 5g

Ingredients:

- 1/2 cup of raw sprouts
- 2 tablespoons of olive oil
- 1/2 cup of kale, shredded
- 1 tablespoon of garlic, minced
- 2 eggs
- 1 tablespoon of turmeric
- 1/4 teaspoon of black pepper

Directions:

- Combine the eggs, black pepper, turmeric, and garlic in a mixing bowl. Sauté the kale in the olive oil for 5 minutes over medium flame, then pour the egg batter into the pan to coat the kale. Cook, stirring frequently, till the eggs are done. Serve with raw sprouts on top.

11. No-Bake Golden Energy Bites
Preparation time: 20 minutes | **Cooking time:** 10 minutes | **Serves:** 4

Per Serving: Calories 376 | Total Fat 36g | Protein 6g | Carbs 9g | Fiber: 2g

Ingredients:

- ½ teaspoon of maple syrup
- 1 teaspoon of coconut oil
- 2 teaspoons of turmeric
- 1 cup of almond butter
- ¾ cup of coconut flakes, unsweetened
- 6 tablespoons of protein powder

Directions:

- In a mixing bowl, combine all of the ingredients until a thick dough forms.
- Spread the dough equally in a pan lined with parchment paper.
- Allow an hour to chill. Remove and cut into pieces.

12. Turmeric Nuggets
Preparation time: 10 minutes | **Cooking time:** 25 minutes | **Serves:** 4

Per Serving: Calories 97 | Total Fat 5g | Protein 7g | Carbs 7g | Fiber: 3g

Ingredients:

- 2 cups of cauliflower florets
- ¼ teaspoon of black pepper
- 2 cups of broccoli florets
- ½ teaspoon of ground turmeric
- 1 cup of carrots, chopped
- ½ cup of almond meal
- 2 egg, pasture-raised

- ¼ teaspoon of salt
- 1 teaspoon of garlic, minced

Directions:
- Preheat the oven to 400°F and line a baking sheet using parchment paper.
- In a food processor, combine all ingredients and pulse till smooth.
- Place a spoonful of the mixture on the baking sheet.
- Bake for around 25 minutes in the oven.

13. Quinoa & Spinach Egg Bites
Preparation time: 10 minutes | **Cooking time:** 20 minutes | **Serves:** 4

Per Serving: Calories 109 | Total Fat 3g | Protein 6g | Carbs 14g | Fiber: 2g

Ingredients:
- 1 tablespoon of chopped parsley
- 1/3 cup of chopped spinach
- 1 cup of cooked quinoa
- Salt and pepper to taste
- 2 large organic pasture-raised eggs

Directions:
- Preheat the oven at 350°F and lightly coat a muffin tray using coconut oil.
- Combine the spinach, quinoa, salt, eggs, parsley, and pepper in a mixing bowl.
- Fill the muffin tins almost to the top with the mixture.
- Bake for around 20 minutes at 350°F.

14. Baked Kale Chips
Preparation time: 10 minutes | **Cooking time:** 20 minutes | **Serves:** 2

Per Serving: Calories 56 | Total Fat 5g | Protein 1g | Carbs 3g | Fiber: 1g

Ingredients:
- 2 teaspoons of olive oil
- 1 bunch of kale, rinsed and dried
- Sea salt and pepper to taste

Directions:
- Preheat the oven at 400°F.
- Rinse and cut the kale into little pieces.
- Spread the greens out on a large baking sheet.
- Season the kale with salt and pepper and drizzle with olive oil.
- Bake for around 10 to 20 minutes. When the kale chips are light and crisp, they are done.

15. Smoked Trout & Mango Wraps
Preparation time: 15 minutes | **Cooking time:** 0 minutes | **Serves:** 4

Per Serving: Calories 108 | Total Fat 3g | Protein 9g | Carbs 13g | Fiber: 1g

Ingredients:

- 4 ounces of trout, smoked, divided
- 1 scallion, sliced, divided
- 4 large green-leaf lettuce leaves, remove the thick stems
- 2 tablespoons of lemon juice, divided
- 1 cup of mango, chopped, divided

Directions:

- Lay the lettuce leaves out on a flat surface. Top each leaf with equal amounts of fish and mango. Drizzle with lemon juice and sprinkle with scallions.
- Wrap the lettuce leaves into a burrito and set them seam-side down on a serving platter.

16. Smoked Turkey–Wrapped Zucchini Sticks

Preparation time: 15 minutes | **Cooking time:** 0 minutes | **Serves:** 4

Per Serving: Calories 137 | Total Fat 3g | Protein 21g | Carbs 6g | Fiber: 2g

Ingredients:

- 1 cup of packed arugula, divided
- 8 thin slices of turkey breast, smoked
- Salt to taste
- 2 zucchinis, quartered lengthwise

Directions:

- Place 1 smoked turkey slice on a work surface. Season with salt and top with 1 zucchini stick and 1/4 cup arugula.
- Wrap the turkey around the veggies and place seam-side down on a plate. Rep with the rest of the ingredients. Serve.

17. Spicy Quinoa

Preparation time: 10 minutes | **Cooking time:** 20 minutes | **Serves:** 4

Per Serving: Calories 286 | Total Fat 13g | Protein 10g | Carbs 32g | Fiber: 6g

Ingredients:

- ½ cup of shredded coconut
- 1 cup of quinoa, rinsed well
- ¼ cup of hemp seeds
- 1 teaspoon of ground cinnamon
- 2 cups of water
- Pinch of salt
- 1 cup of fresh berries of your choice, divided
- 2 tablespoons of flaxseed
- ¼ cup of chopped hazelnuts
- 1 teaspoon of vanilla extract

Directions:

- Combine the quinoa and water in a medium saucepan over a high flame.

- Bring to boil, then reduce to a low flame and cook for 15 to 20 minutes, or till the quinoa is tender (it should double or triple in bulk, similar to couscous, and be somewhat transparent).
- Combine the cinnamon, coconut, vanilla, hemp seeds, flaxseed, and salt in a mixing bowl.
- Divide the quinoa among four bowls and top with 1/4 cup berries and 1 tbsp. hazelnuts for each serving.

18. Herb Scramble with Sautéed Cherry Tomatoes
Preparation time: 5 minutes | **Cooking time:** 10 minutes | **Serves:** 2

Per Serving: Calories 310 | Total Fat 26g | Protein 13g | Carbs 10g | Fiber: 6g

Ingredients:

- 1 cup of cherry tomatoes, halved
- ½ avocado, sliced
- 4 eggs
- 1 tablespoon of extra-virgin olive oil
- 2 teaspoons of chopped fresh oregano
- ½ garlic clove, sliced

Directions:

- In a medium mixing bowl, whisk together the eggs and oregano.
- Heat a large-sized skillet on a medium-high flame. Add the olive oil once the pan is heated.
- Pour the eggs into the skillet and scramble them using a heat-resistant spatula or wooden spoon. Place the eggs in a serving dish.
- Sauté the cherry tomatoes and garlic in the pan for about 2 minutes. Place the tomatoes on top of the eggs and garnish with the avocado slices.

19. Blueberry Breakfast Blend
Preparation time: 5 minutes | **Cooking time:** 0 minutes | **Serves:** 1

Per Serving: Calories 260 | Total Fat 8g | Protein 13g | Carbs 39g | Fiber: 7g

Ingredients:

- 1 tablespoon of chia seeds
- 1/ 3 teaspoon of turmeric
- 1 cup of water
- ¾ cup of fresh blueberries
- 1 cup of fresh pineapple chunks
- ½ cup of spinach
- 1 tablespoon of lemon juice

Directions:

- In a blender, combine all of the ingredients. Blend till the mixture is smooth.

20. Green Smoothie Bowl
Preparation time: 10 minutes | **Cooking time:** 0 minutes | **Serves:** 2

Per Serving: Calories 352 | Total Fat 18g | Protein 8g | Carbs 35g | Fiber: 2g

Ingredients:

- ¼ cup of almonds, toasted and chopped
- 1 cup of fresh strawberries, hulled
- ¼ of ripe avocado, peeled, pitted, and chopped
- 1 cup of fresh spinach
- 2 medium ripe bananas, frozen and sliced
- 1 cup of fresh kale, trimmed
- 1½ cups of unsweetened almond milk
- 1 tablespoon of flaxseed meal
- ¼ cup of unsweetened shredded coconut

Directions:

- Except for the almonds and coconut, combine all ingredients in a high-speed blender. Blend till smoothen.
- Transfer the purée to serving bowls and top with almonds and coconut.

21. Zucchini Chips

Preparation time: 10 minutes | **Cooking time:** 15 minutes | **Serves:** 2

Per Serving: Calories 40 | Total Fat 2g | Protein 1g | Carbs 1g | Fiber: 0.1g

Ingredients:

- 1/8 teaspoon of ground cumin
- 1 medium zucchini, cut into thin slices
- 1/8 teaspoon of ground turmeric
- 2 teaspoons of olive oil
- Salt, to taste

Directions:

- Preheat the oven at 400°F. 2 baking sheets should be lined with parchment paper.
- Toss all ingredients in a large mixing dish to coat well.
- Place a single layer of the mixture on prepared baking sheets.
- Bake for around 10 to 15 minutes.
- Serve right away.

22. Quinoa & Seeds Crackers

Preparation time: 10 minutes | **Cooking time:** 20 minutes | **Serves:** 2

Per Serving: Calories 34 | Total Fat 2g | Protein 1g | Carbs 2g | Fiber: 0.6g

Ingredients:

- 4 tablespoons of water
- 1 1/2 teaspoons of ground turmeric
- 2 tablespoons of chia seeds
- 2 tablespoons of quinoa flour
- Pinch of ground cinnamon
- 4 tablespoons of sunflower seeds
- Salt, to taste

Directions:

- Preheat the oven at 345°F. Using parchment paper, line a baking sheet.
- Soak the chia seeds in water for about a quarter-hour in a bowl.
- After fifteen minutes, add the other ingredients and well combine.
- Spread the mixture onto the baking sheet that has been prepared.
- Bake for around 20 minutes.

23. Green Tea and Pear Smoothie
Preparation time: 10 minutes | **Cooking time:** 0 minutes | **Serves:** 2

Per Serving: Calories 208 | Total Fat 2g | Protein 1g | Carbs 41g | Fiber: 7g

Ingredients:

- 1 (one-inch) piece of fresh ginger, peeled and roughly chopped
- 2 cups of strongly brewed green tea
- 1 cup of unsweetened almond milk
- 2 tablespoons of honey
- 1 cup of crushed ice
- 2 pears, peeled, cored and chopped

Directions:

- Combine the green tea, almond milk, pears, ginger, honey, and ice in a blender. Blend till completely smooth.

24. Pineapple Sticks
Preparation time: 10 minutes | **Cooking time:** 0 minutes | **Serves:** 4

Per Serving: Calories 65 | Total Fat 3g | Protein 0g | Carbs 10g | Fiber: 1g

Ingredients:

- ¾ cup of coconut, shredded and toasted
- 4 (3x1-inch) new pineapple pieces
- ¼ cup of fresh pineapple or orange juice

Directions:

- Wax paper should be used to line a baking pan.
- Place pineapple juice in a small dish.
- Squeeze the pineapple into another shallow dish.
- Insert 1 wooden skewer through the narrow end of each pineapple piece.
- Each pineapple piece should be dipped in juice and then uniformly coated with coconut.
- Arrange the pineapple sticks in a single layer on a prepared baking sheet.
- Cover and place in the freezer for 1-2 hours.

25. Roasted Cashews
Preparation time: 10 minutes | **Cooking time:** 25 minutes | **Serves:** 4

Per Serving: Calories 200 | Total Fat 17g | Protein 4g | Carbs 11g | Fiber: 1g

Ingredients:

- 1 tablespoon of freshly squeezed lemon juice
- 1 1/2 cups of cashews
- 1 teaspoon of smoked paprika
- 2 teaspoons of raw honey
- ½ teaspoon of chili flakes
- 1 teaspoon of olive oil
- Salt, to taste

Directions:
- Preheat the oven at 350°F. Using parchment paper, line a baking dish.
- Toss all ingredients inside a bowl to coat well.
- Place the cashew mixture in a single layer in the prepared baking dish.
- Roast for about 20 minutes, flipping once halfway through roasting.
- Remove from the oven and set aside to completely cool before serving.
- These roasted cashews can be stored in an airtight jar.

26. Fruity Bowl
Preparation time: 10 minutes | **Cooking time:** 0 minutes | **Serves:** 2

Per Serving: Calories 211 | Total Fat 3g | Protein 4g | Carbs 49g | Fiber: 1g

Ingredients:
- 2 tablespoons of Chia seeds
- 1 large apple, peeled, cored, and chopped
- 2 cups of frozen cherries, pitted
- 4 dates, pitted and chopped
- A cup of fresh cherries pitted

Directions:
- Blend frozen cherries and dates in a high-speed blender till smooth.
- In a mixing dish, combine the chopped apple, fresh cherries, and Chia seeds.
- Stir in the cherry sauce to the purée and mix.
- Before serving, cover and chill them overnight.

27. Coconut & Banana Cookies
Preparation time: 10 minutes | **Cooking time:** 25 minutes | **Serves:** 4

Per Serving: Calories 370 | Total Fat 4g | Protein 33g | Carbs 28g | Fiber: 11g

Ingredients:
- ½ teaspoon of ground cinnamon
- 1 cup of unsweetened coconut, shredded
- Pinch of salt to taste
- 2 medium bananas, peeled
- Freshly ground black pepper
- ½ teaspoon of ground turmeric

Directions:

- Preheat the oven at 350°F. Line a cookie sheet using parchment paper that has been gently oiled.
- Combine all of the ingredients in a mixer and pulse till dough-like consistency forms.
- Form little balls from the mixture and place them in a single layer on a prepared cookie sheet.
- Press your fingers along the balls to make the cookies.
- Bake for 15 to 20 minutes or till golden brown.

28. Apple Bruschetta with Almonds and Blackberries
Preparation time: 15 minutes | **Cooking time:** 0 minutes | **Serves:** 2

Per Serving: Calories 56 | Total Fat 2g | Protein 2g | Carbs 9g | Fiber: 11g

Ingredients:

- ¼ cup of blackberries, thawed, lightly mashed
- 1 apple, sliced into ¼-inch thick half-moons
- ½ teaspoon of fresh lemon juice
- Sea salt to taste
- 1/8 cup of almond slivers, toasted

Directions:

- Apple slices should be sprinkled with lemon juice. Place them on a tray lined using parchment paper.
- Place a small amount of mashed berries on top of each slice. Top with the desired amount of almond slivers.
- Season the "bruschetta" with sea salt just before serving.

29. Green Apple and Spinach Smoothie
Preparation time: 10 minutes | **Cooking time:** 0 minutes | **Serves:** 1

Per Serving: Calories 176 | Total Fat 1g | Protein 2g | Carbs 41g | Fiber: 6g

Ingredients:

- ½ teaspoon of raw honey or pure maple syrup
- ½ cup of coconut water
- 1 cup of spinach
- ¼ lemon, seeded
- 1 green apple, cored, seeded, and quartered
- Ice (optional)
- ½ cucumber peeled and seeded

Directions:

- Blend together the lemon, coconut water, honey, apple, spinach, cucumber, and ice (if using) inside a blender. Blend till completely smooth.

30. Ginger Date Bars
Preparation time: 10 minutes | **Cooking time:** 20 minutes | **Serves:** 4

Per Serving: Calories 45 | Total Fat 0.3g | Protein 0.5g | Carbs 11g | Fiber: 1g

Ingredients:

- ¼ cup of almond milk
- 1 cup of almonds, soaked in water overnight, then drained
- 1 teaspoon of ground ginger
- ¾ cup of pitted dates

Directions:

- Preheat the oven at 350°F.
- In a food processor, blend the almonds. Pulse till a thick dough forms.
- Line a baking dish using parchment paper and press the dough into it. Place aside.
- In a food processor, add the remaining ingredients for the date mix. Blend till smooth.
- Fill the almond crust with the date mixture. Bake for around 20 minutes at 350°F. Allow to cool before slicing.

Chapter 8: Light Lunches and Salads

1. Cabbage Orange Salad with Citrusy Vinaigrette
Preparation time: 10 minutes | **Cooking time:** 0 minutes | **Serves:** 4

Per Serving: Calories 70 | Total Fat 0.1g | Protein 1g | Carbs 14g | Fiber: 3g

Ingredients:

- 1 teaspoon of lemon juice
- 1/4 teaspoon of salt
- 1 teaspoon of orange zest, grated
- 1 1/2 tablespoons of vegetable stock, reduced-sodium
- 1 tablespoon of fresh orange juice
- 1/2 teaspoon of cider vinegar
- 2 cups red cabbage, shredded
- Freshly ground pepper
- 1/2 fennel bulb, sliced thinly
- 2 teaspoons of olive oil
- 1/2 teaspoon of raspberry vinegar
- 1 orange, peeled, cut into pieces
- 1/2 teaspoon of balsamic vinegar
- 1 tablespoon of honey

Directions:

- Inside a mixing bowl, combine the lemon juice, balsamic vinegar, orange zest, cider vinegar, salt and pepper, orange juice, broth, oil, honey, and raspberry.
- Add fennel, oranges, and cabbage. To coat, mix.

2. Moroccan Lentil Soup
Preparation time: 10 minutes | **Cooking time:** 45 minutes | **Serves:** 4

Per Serving: Calories 238 | Total Fat 7g | Protein 14g | Carbs 32g | Fiber: 6.2g

Ingredients:

- 6 cups of vegetable broth, low salt
- 1 cup of red lentils, dry, rinsed
- 28 ounces of whole tomatoes, canned, mashed with juice
- 1 teaspoon of cinnamon
- 1 (15-ounces) can of chickpeas, drain and rinse
- 1 teaspoon of salt
- ½ cup of cilantro, chopped
- 2 garlic
- 1 teaspoon of black pepper
- 2 tablespoons of olive oil
- 1 onion, yellow, chopped

- 2 celery stalks finely chopped
- 1 teaspoon of turmeric
- 2 teaspoons of paprika
- ½ cup of chopped parsley
- 2 tablespoons of ginger, minced
- 2 Carrots

Directions:

- Cook garlic, carrots, celery, ginger, and onion for 10 minutes in heated oil, stirring frequently.
- Cook for 5 minutes to thoroughly combine the paprika, pepper, cinnamon, salt, and turmeric.
- Mix in the broth and tomatoes thoroughly. Reduce the flame to low and add the cilantro, parsley, chickpeas, and lentils. Allow the soup to simmer for around 30 minutes.

3. Coconut Mushroom Soup
Preparation time: 10 minutes | **Cooking time:** 15 minutes | **Serves:** 3

Per Serving: Calories 143 | Total Fat 14g | Protein 2g | Carbs 4g | Fiber: 1g

Ingredients:

- 1 cup of cremini mushrooms, chopped
- 1 tablespoon of coconut oil
- ½ cup canned coconut milk
- 1 tablespoon of ground ginger
- ½ teaspoon of turmeric
- Sea salt to taste
- 2 ½ cups of water

Directions:

- Inside a large pot, heat the coconut oil over medium flame and add the mushrooms. Cook for around 3-4 minutes.
- Bring the remaining ingredients to a gentle boil. Allow it to simmer for 5 minutes.
- Divide among three soup bowls and serve.

4. Anti-Inflammatory Kale Salad
Preparation time: 10 minutes | **Cooking time:** 0 minutes | **Serves:** 1

Per Serving: Calories 477 | Total Fat 33g | Protein 6g | Carbs 48g | Fiber: 7g

Ingredients:

- ½ cup of pitted cherries, halved
- 1 cup of fresh kale
- 2 tablespoons of olive oil
- ½ cup of blueberries
- Juice of 1 lemon
- ¼ cup of dried cranberries
- 1 tablespoon of sesame seeds

Directions:

- Toss the kale in the dressing after whisking together the olive oil and lemon juice.
- Toss the kale leaves with the fresh blueberries, cherries, and cranberries in a large salad bowl.
- Sesame seeds should be sprinkled on top.

5. Spinach Bean Salad
Preparation time: 10 minutes | **Cooking time:** 5 minutes | **Serves:** 1

Per Serving: Calories 274 | Total Fat 15g | Protein 9g | Carbs 26g | Fiber: 8g

Ingredients:
- 1 tablespoon of olive oil
- ½ cup of canned garbanzo beans
- 1 cup of fresh spinach
- ¼ cup of canned black beans
- 2 tablespoons of organic balsamic vinaigrette
- ½ cup of cremini mushrooms

Directions:
- Cook the cremini mushrooms in the olive oil for 5 minutes, or till gently browned, over a medium flame.
- To make the salad, place the fresh spinach on a platter and top with the beans, mushrooms, and balsamic vinaigrette.

6. Smashed Chickpea Avocado Salad Sandwich with Cranberries
Preparation time: 10 minutes | **Cooking time:** 10 minutes | **Serves:** 2

Per Serving: Calories 405 | Total Fat 15g | Protein 12g | Carbs 24g | Fiber: 17g

Ingredients:
- 2 teaspoons of lemon juice, squeezed
- Arugula, spinach, or red onion to top
- 4 slices of whole-wheat bread
- Black pepper & salt
- 1 large ripe avocado
- ¼ cup of cranberries, dried
- 1 can of chickpeas, rinsed & drained

Directions:
- In a medium-sized mixing bowl, mash the chickpeas using a large fork. Add the avocado and mash again with the same fork till absolutely smooth; don't worry if it has some chunky pieces.
- Season with pepper and salt to taste after adding the cranberries and lemon juice. Refrigerate until ready to serve.
- To serve, toast the bread and spread about 1/2 of the chickpea avocado salad on one slice. Serve with arugula, spinach, or red onion on top. Top with another toasted piece and split in half. Serve right away and enjoy.

7. Salmon Salad
Preparation time: 10 minutes | **Cooking time:** 0 minutes | **Serves:** 1

Per Serving: Calories 553 | Total Fat 37g | Protein 48g | Carbs 24g | Fiber: 17g

Ingredients:

- 1 teaspoon of Dijon mustard
- 1 cup of organic arugula
- 1 teaspoon of sea salt
- 1 can of wild-caught salmon
- ½ of an avocado, sliced
- 1 tablespoon of olive oil

Directions:

- To make the dressing, whisk together the Dijon mustard, olive oil, and sea salt in a mixing bowl. Place aside.
- Assemble the salad with the arugula as the foundation and the salmon and avocado slices on top.
- Drizzle the dressing on top.

8. Sweet Potato Patties

Preparation time: 10 minutes | **Cooking time:** 10 minutes | **Serves:** 4

Per Serving: Calories 359 | Total Fat 5g | Protein 8g | Carbs 42g | Fiber: 10g

Ingredients:

- 4 tablespoons of coconut oil for cooking
- 2 ½ cups of sweet potato, peeled & shredded
- ½ cup of white onion, chopped
- 1 large organic pasture-raised egg, beaten
- 1/3 cup of coconut flour
- Salt and pepper to taste

Directions:

- In a large mixing dish, combine the sweet potato and flour. Mix in the onion and the egg.
- Form the sweet potato mixture into four balls, each into a tiny patty.
- Melt 3 to 4 tablespoons of coconut oil in a saucepan over medium flame.
- Cook each patty for 3 minutes on each side or till golden brown.
- For the ultimate anti-inflammatory lunch, serve with a side salad.

9. Tuscany Vegetable Soup

Preparation time: 15 minutes | **Cooking time:** 30 minutes | **Serves:** 4

Per Serving: Calories 225 | Total Fat 6g | Protein 17g | Carbs 12g | Fiber: 10g

Ingredients:

- 1 medium yellow onion, diced
- 1 medium zucchini, peeled and chopped
- 1/4 cup of celery, chopped
- Parsley, fresh chopped for garnishing
- 1/4 cup of carrot
- 2 tablespoons of tomato paste

- 1 cup of kale, chopped
- 3 tablespoons of olive oil
- 1 tomato, large diced small
- ½ teaspoon of salt
- 1 teaspoon of black pepper
- 3 cups of vegetable broth
- 1 tablespoon of basil, finely chopped
- 2 tablespoons of garlic, minced

Directions:

- In a big pan, heat the olive oil and fry the garlic and onion. Cook for 10 minutes, stirring regularly, after adding the celery, zucchini, and carrots. Cook for 2 minutes more after adding salt, pepper, and tomatoes.
- After adding the vegetable broth and tomato paste, bring to boil. Reduce the flame to low and let the mixture simmer for fifteen minutes.
- Remove the soup from the flame and set aside for 10 minutes after adding the basil and parsley. Serve the soup garnished with fresh parsley.

10. Cabbage Soup

Preparation time: 15 minutes | **Cooking time:** 45 minutes | **Serves:** 4

Per Serving: Calories 90 | Total Fat 1g | Protein 5g | Carbs 20g | Fiber: 5g

Ingredients:

- 1 tablespoon of thyme
- 2 cups of green cabbage
- ½ cup of mushrooms
- 2 carrots
- 1 medium onion
- Pepper to taste
- 2 cups of vegetable stock
- 1 cup of water
- Sea salt to taste
- 1 tablespoon of rosemary

Directions:

- Place all of the vegetables in a pot with the vegetable stock.
- Add water and cook for 15-20 minutes on medium flame. Allow to come to boil, then reduce to a low flame and add the thyme and rosemary, cooking for around 25 minutes more.
- Season the soup using salt and pepper to taste.
- Serve hot & enjoy.

11. Fish Sticks with Avocado Dipping Sauce

Preparation time: 15 minutes | **Cooking time:** 5 minutes | **Serves:** 4

Per Serving: Calories 483 | Total Fat 20g | Protein 14g | Carbs 14g | Fiber: 6g

Ingredients:

For the avocado dipping sauce:

- 2 tablespoons of fresh cilantro leaves
- ¼ cup of lime juice
- Dash ground cumin
- 2 tablespoons of olive oil
- 1 teaspoon of salt
- 2 avocados
- 1 teaspoon of garlic powder
- Black pepper

For the fish sticks:

- ¼ cup of coconut oil
- 1 teaspoon of salt
- ½ teaspoon of paprika
- 1 pound of cod fillets, cut into four-inch-long, one-inch-thick strips
- ¼ teaspoon of black pepper
- 3 eggs
- 1 ½ cups of almond flour
- Juice of 1 lemon

Directions:

- Blend the avocados, lime juice, garlic powder, cilantro, olive oil, salt, and cumin in a food processor till smooth and season with pepper.
- In a small shallow dish, combine the almond flour, paprika, salt, and pepper. In another small shallow dish, whisk the eggs.
- Dip the fish sticks until completely coated in the egg and almond flour mixture.
- Heat the coconut oil in a suitable skillet over a medium-high flame.
- Place the fish sticks in the skillet one at a time. Cook for approximately 2 minutes on each side till gently browned. Divide them between two plates.
- Sprinkle with lemon juice and serve alongside the avocado dipping sauce.

12. Buckwheat and Onion Soup

Preparation time: 15 minutes | **Cooking time:** 20 minutes | **Serves:** 3

Per Serving: Calories 389 | Total Fat 18g | Protein 8g | Carbs 39g | Fiber: 6g

Ingredients:

- 2 cups of unsweetened coconut milk
- 1 pinch of salt
- 2 sweet potatoes
- 1/2 cup of buckwheat
- 1 shallot
- 2 cups of red onions
- 1 tablespoon of thyme

- 1 pinch of cayenne pepper
- 3 cups of low sodium vegetable broth
- 1 clove of garlic
- 3 tablespoons of olive oil
- 1 pinch of salt

Directions:

- Chop the garlic, onions, and shallots together.
- Brown the diced potatoes in a pan with the chopped onions and garlic for 5 minutes before adding the thyme.
- Add the coconut milk, salt, and pepper, and vegetable broth, and bring to boil. Add the buckwheat and cook for about 20 minutes over moderate flame.
- The soup can be consumed as it is or pureed.

13. Sweet Potato Quinoa
Preparation time: 10 minutes | **Cooking time:** 25 minutes | **Serves:** 4

Per Serving: Calories 188 | Total Fat 8g | Protein 31g | Carbs 26g | Fiber: 5g

Ingredients:

- 1 cup of quinoa
- 2 sweet potatoes
- ¼ teaspoon of ground black pepper
- 2 cups of kale
- ¼ teaspoon of salt
- 2 cups of vegetable broth
- 1 tablespoon of apple cider vinegar
- 2 tablespoons of olive oil
- 1 tablespoon of garlic, minced
- 2 tablespoons of fresh chervil

Directions:

- Remove the ends of the sweet potatoes, peel them, and dice them into 1/4-inch pieces.
- In a skillet, combine the olive oil and sweet potatoes. Cook for 2 minutes over medium-high flame.
- Mix in the quinoa, garlic, salt, apple cider vinegar, and pepper. Cook for an additional 2 minutes.
- Reduce the flame to low and add the vegetable broth. Stir everything together, then covers and cook for 12 minutes.
- Remove the lid and mix in the kale and chervil. Cook for 3 minutes, or till all of the ingredients are soft and well blended, before serving.

14. Stuffed Sweet Potatoes
Preparation time: 15 minutes | **Cooking time:** 55 minutes | **Serves:** 4

Per Serving: Calories 267 | Total Fat 8g | Protein 9g | Carbs 42g | Fiber: 7g

Ingredients:

- ½ white onion, minced

- 4 sweet potatoes
- 1 can (15 ounces) of black beans
- 1 tablespoon of garlic
- ¼ cup of sundried tomatoes, halved
- 1 teaspoon of salt
- 2 tablespoons of olive oil
- 1 teaspoon of clove

Directions:

- Preheat the oven at 350°F.
- Line a baking sheet using foil and place the sweet potatoes on top. Bake for 45 minutes with 1 tablespoon of olive oil drizzled over sweet potatoes.
- In a skillet, heat 1 tablespoon olive oil on medium flame and sauté onion for 4 minutes. Cook for additional 2 minutes, stirring constantly, after adding the garlic.
- Cook until the sundried tomatoes and black beans are warmed through after adding them, about 2 minutes.
- Cut the sweet potatoes lengthwise and pull them apart to lay them flat. Top with onions, beans, garlic, and tomatoes. Serve with a pinch of clove and salt.

15. Avocado & Grapefruit Salad
Preparation time: 10 minutes | **Cooking time:** 0 minutes | **Serves:** 2

Per Serving: Calories 228 | Total Fat 20g | Protein 3g | Carbs 42g | Fiber: 14g

Ingredients:

- 1 avocado
- 1/2 teaspoon of dried mint
- 1 grapefruit
- ½ teaspoon of sea salt

Directions:

- Grapefruit and avocado should be peeled and sliced into pieces.
- Save the avocado shells for later use as bowls.
- Toss the avocado and grapefruit with the sea salt and mint. Serve this salad as a side dish in the reserved avocado "bowls."

16. White Bean & Tuna Salad
Preparation time: 10 minutes | **Cooking time:** 0 minutes | **Serves:** 4

Per Serving: Calories 373 | Total Fat 19g | Protein 29g | Carbs 28g | Fiber: 14g

Ingredients:

- ½ cup of pitted Kalamata olives
- 4 cups of arugula
- 2 tablespoons of olive oil
- 1 (15-ounce) can of white beans
- ½ pint of cherry tomatoes halved

- 2 (5-ounces) cans of flaked white tuna
- ½ red onion, chopped
- ¼ cup of extra-virgin olive oil
- 2 tablespoons of lemon juice, freshly squeezed
- Salt & pepper to taste

Directions:

- Combine the arugula, olive oil, tuna, white beans, onion, tomatoes, olives, and lemon juice in a mixing bowl. Season using salt and pepper to taste.
- Drizzle with olive oil and serve.

17. Mediterranean Chopped Salad
Preparation time: 10 minutes | **Cooking time:** 0 minutes | **Serves:** 2

Per Serving: Calories 194 | Total Fat 14g | Protein 4g | Carbs 15g | Fiber: 9g

Ingredients:

- 2 cups of packed spinach
- 3 large tomatoes, diced
- 1 bunch of radishes, sliced thin
- 2 scallions, sliced
- 1 tablespoon of apple cider vinegar
- 2 garlic cloves, minced
- 1 tablespoon of fresh mint, chopped
- 1 cup of almond yogurt
- ¼ cup of extra-virgin olive oil
- 1 tablespoon of fresh parsley, chopped
- 3 tablespoons of lemon juice, freshly squeezed
- 1 English cucumber, peeled and diced
- Salt, & pepper to taste
- 1 tablespoon of sumac

Directions:

- Toss together the spinach, parsley, pepper, tomatoes, radishes, cider vinegar, cucumber, scallions, salt, olive oil, garlic, mint, yogurt, lemon juice, and sumac in a large mixing dish. To mix, toss everything together.

18. Mushrooms in Broth
Preparation time: 15 minutes | **Cooking time:** 10 minutes | **Serves:** 4

Per Serving: Calories 111 | Total Fat 5g | Protein 9g | Carbs 9g | Fiber: 4g

Ingredients:

- 2 tablespoons of fresh tarragon, chopped
- 1 tablespoon of extra-virgin olive oil
- Salt & pepper to taste
- 1 onion, halved, sliced thinly

- 3 garlic cloves, sliced
- 1 pound of mushrooms, sliced
- 4 cups of vegetable broth
- 1 celery stalk, chopped

Directions:

- Warm the olive oil in a pot over a high flame.
- Add the garlic, onion, and celery. Cook for 3 minutes.
- Add the salt, mushrooms, and pepper. Cook for another 5 to 10 minutes.
- Bring the soup to a boil with the veggie broth. Reduce the flame to a gentle simmer. Cook for an additional 5 minutes.
- Serve with the tarragon stirred in.

19. Coconut Fish Stew

Preparation time: 15 minutes | **Cooking time:** 15 minutes | **Serves:** 4

Per Serving: Calories 80 | Total Fat 43g | Protein 46g | Carbs 13g | Fiber: 8g

Ingredients:

- ½ cup of slivered scallions
- 2 tablespoons of coconut oil
- 1 white onion, sliced
- 2 garlic cloves, sliced
- 1 (13.5-ounce) can of coconut milk
- 2 zucchinis, sliced
- 1 ½ pounds of firm white fish fillet, cut into cubes
- 1 (4-inch) piece of lemongrass, bruised
- 3 tablespoons of lemon juice, freshly squeezed
- Salt & white pepper, to taste
- ¼ cup of cilantro, chopped

Directions:

- Melt the coconut oil in a saucepan on medium flame.
- Add the garlic, onion, and zucchini. Cook for around 5 minutes.
- To the pot, add the fish, salt, lemongrass, coconut milk, and white pepper. Bring to boil, then reduce to a low flame and continue to cook for 5 minutes. Take out the lemongrass.
- Stir in the lemon juice and garnish with scallions and cilantro. Serve.

20. Mixed Berry Salad with Ginger

Preparation time: 15 minutes | **Cooking time:** 0 minutes | **Serves:** 4

Per Serving: Calories 75 | Total Fat 1g | Protein 1g | Carbs 18g | Fiber: 5g

Ingredients:

- 1 cup of fresh blueberries
- 1 cup of fresh strawberries
- 1 tablespoon of grated fresh ginger

- Zest of 1 orange
- 1 cup of fresh raspberries
- Juice of 1 orange

Directions:

- In a medium mixing dish, combine the blueberries, orange zest, raspberries, strawberries, ginger, and orange juice.

Chapter 9: Main Dishes

1. Chicken and Broccoli

Preparation time: 10 minutes | **Cooking time:** 10 minutes | **Serves:** 4

Per Serving: Calories 345 | Total Fat 14g | Protein 18g | Carbs 41g | Fiber: 3g

Ingredients:

- 3 tablespoons of extra-virgin olive oil
- ⅛ teaspoon of black pepper
- 1 ½ pounds of boneless and skinless chicken breasts, make bite-size chunks
- ½ onion, chopped
- ½ teaspoon of sea salt
- 3 garlic cloves, minced
- 1 ½ cups of broccoli florets or chopped broccoli stems
- 2 cups of cooked brown rice

Directions:

- Heat the olive oil in a large nonstick skillet on medium-high flame till it shimmers.
- Now add the chicken, broccoli, onion, salt, and pepper. Cook, tossing periodically, for about 7 minutes or till the chicken is done.
- Mix in the garlic. Cook for 30 seconds while constantly stirring.
- To serve, toss with the brown rice.

2. Trout with Sweet-and-Sour Chard

Preparation time: 10 minutes | **Cooking time:** 15 minutes | **Serves:** 4

Per Serving: Calories 231 | Total Fat 10g | Protein 24g | Carbs 13g | Fiber: 6g

Ingredients:

- 2 garlic cloves, minced
- 1 tablespoon of apple cider vinegar
- 4 boneless trout fillets
- Salt & pepper to taste
- 1 tablespoon of extra-virgin olive oil
- ¼ cup of golden raisins
- 1 onion, chopped
- 2 bunches of chard, sliced
- ½ cup of vegetable broth

Directions:

- Preheat the oven at 375°F.
- Season the trout well using salt and pepper.
- Heat the olive oil in an ovenproof pan. Mix in the onion and garlic. Sauté for 3 minutes, then add the chard and cook for another 2 minutes.
- Pour in the cider vinegar, raisins, and broth. On top, arrange the fish fillets. Place the pan in a preheated oven for 10 minutes or till the fish is cooked.

3. Sweet Potato Curry with Spinach

Preparation time: 10 minutes | **Cooking time:** 25 minutes | **Serves:** 4

Per Serving: Calories 314 | Total Fat 11g | Protein 8g | Carbs 50g | Fiber: 9g

Ingredients:

- 2 tablespoons of extra-virgin olive oil
- 3 cups of vegetable broth, no-salt-added
- 1/2 teaspoon of sea salt
- 1 chopped onion
- 4 cups of fresh baby spinach
- 2 tablespoons of curry powder
- 1/8 teaspoon of black pepper
- 4 cups of cubed & peeled sweet potato
- 1 cup of lite coconut milk

Directions:

- Heat the olive oil in a big pot on medium-high flame till it shimmers.
- Mix in the onion. Cook for 5 minutes, stirring occasionally, till tender.
- Combine the sweet potato, salt, spinach, vegetable broth, curry powder, coconut milk, and pepper. Bring to the boil, then lower to a medium flame. Cook, stirring periodically, for about 15 minutes, till the sweet potatoes are tender.

4. Superfood Bowl

Preparation time: 10 minutes | **Cooking time:** 40 minutes | **Serves:** 2

Per Serving: Calories 224 | Total Fat 14g | Protein 12g | Carbs 15g | Fiber: 5g

Ingredients:

- 1 tablespoon of tahini dressing
- ¼ cup of uncooked quinoa rinsed
- ½ cup of canned black beans
- ¼ avocado
- 2 large stalks of kale
- ½ cup of lentils
- ½ sweet potato, peeled & cubed
- Himalayan sea salt to taste
- ½ cup of cauliflower

Directions:

- First, bake the sweet potato at 375°F for around 25 minutes, rotating once.
- While the potatoes are in the oven, you can start boiling some quinoa by bringing half a cup of dry quinoa and a quarter cup of water to boil. Add more water if necessary and simmer for 20 minutes.
- The lentils need to be washed and then cooked in a pot of boiling water. Lentils need to be boiled for 25 minutes.
- Cook the kale in a skillet, then steam the cauliflower and cut up 1 avocado.

- After the quinoa has finished cooking, transfer it to a serving bowl and top it with the aforementioned vegetables and lentils.
- Spread tahini on top and season with salt to taste.

5. Tomato Asparagus Frittata
Preparation time: 10 minutes | **Cooking time:** 15 minutes | **Serves:** 4

Per Serving: Calories 224 | Total Fat 14g | Protein 12g | Carbs 15g | Fiber: 5g

Ingredients:

- 2 tablespoons of extra-virgin olive oil
- 10 cherry tomatoes
- 1/2 teaspoon of sea salt
- 6 eggs
- 1/8 teaspoon of black pepper
- 10 asparagus spears, trimmed
- 1 tablespoon of chopped fresh thyme

Directions:

- Turn on the oven broiler to high.
- Heat the olive oil in a large ovenproof skillet on medium-high flame till it shimmers.
- Stir in the asparagus. Cook, stirring periodically, for 5 minutes.
- Mix in the tomatoes. Cook, stirring periodically, for 3 minutes.
- Inside a medium mixing bowl, combine the thyme, eggs, salt, and pepper. Pour over the tomatoes and the asparagus, swirling them around so they are properly distributed in the pan.
- Turn the flame down to medium. Cook the eggs for 3 minutes or till they are set around the edges. Pull the eggs away from the skillet's sides with a rubber spatula and tilt the pan to allow the raw eggs to run into the edges. Cook for 3 minutes or till the edges re-set.
- Place the pan under the broiler for 3 to 5 minutes or until puffed and brown. To serve, cut into wedges.

6. Braised Bok Choy with Shiitake Mushrooms
Preparation time: 10 minutes | **Cooking time:** 15 minutes | **Serves:** 4

Per Serving: Calories 285 | Total Fat 8g | Protein 26g | Carbs 43g | Fiber: 18g

Ingredients:

- 1 tablespoon of coconut aminos
- 1 tablespoon of coconut oil
- 8 baby bok choy, halved lengthwise
- 1 tablespoon of toasted sesame seeds
- ½ cup of water
- Freshly ground black pepper
- 1 cup of shiitake mushrooms, stemmed, thinly sliced
- Salt
- 1 scallion, thinly sliced

Directions:

- Melt the coconut oil in a large-sized saucepan on high flame. Bok choy should be added in a single layer.
- To the pan, add the coconut aminos, water, and mushrooms. Cook the vegetables, covered, for 5 to 10 minutes or till the bok choy is soft.
- Take the pan off the flame. Season using salt and pepper to taste.
- Place the bok choy and mushrooms on a serving platter and top with the scallions and sesame seeds.

7. Butternut Squash and Spinach Gratin with Lentils

Preparation time: 15 minutes | **Cooking time:** 25 minutes | **Serves:** 4

Per Serving: Calories 502 | Total Fat 37g | Protein 20g | Carbs 47g | Fiber: 16g

Ingredients:

- 1 small butternut squash, peeled, and seeded, make ½-inch cubes
- 1 (13.5-ounce) can of coconut milk
- 2 tablespoons of chopped fresh sage
- 1 tablespoon of coconut oil
- ¼ cup of chopped fresh parsley
- 2 garlic cloves, minced
- 1 teaspoon of salt
- ½ teaspoon of ground black pepper
- 1 onion, peeled and chopped
- 1½ or 2 cups of vegetable broth
- 4 cups of packed spinach
- 1 (15-ounce) can of lentils, drained and rinsed
- ½ cup of chopped toasted walnuts

Directions:

- Preheat your oven at 375°F.
- Melt the coconut oil in a large-sized ovenproof skillet on high flame. Mix in the onion and garlic. Cook for 3 minutes.
- Add the spinach, butternut squash, salt, and pepper. Cook for another 3 minutes.
- Add the coconut milk and enough vegetable broth to cover the squash. Bring the liquid to a rolling boil.
- Add the parsley, lentils, and sage. To combine, stir everything together.
- Transfer to the oven and bake the casserole in the oven for 15 to 20 minutes or until the squash is soft.
- Place the casserole in a serving dish and top with the walnuts.

8. Eggplant and Tomato Stew

Preparation time: 10 minutes | **Cooking time:** 25 minutes | **Serves:** 3

Per Serving: Calories 210 | Total Fat 5g | Protein 8g | Carbs 14g | Fiber: 5g

Ingredients:

- 1 teaspoon of ground cumin
- 2 big tomatoes, chopped

- 1 cup of tomato paste
- A pinch of cayenne pepper
- 1 yellow onion, chopped
- A pinch of salt and black pepper
- 1 eggplant, chopped
- ½ cup of vegetable stock

Directions:

- Heat the stock in a small saucepan on medium flame. Toss in the tomato paste, cayenne pepper, tomatoes, salt, eggplant, pepper, and onion. Stir well, bring to a simmer, cover, and cook for 25 minutes. Serve in individual bowls. Enjoy!

9. Salmon with Salsa
Preparation time: 10 minutes | **Cooking time:** 15 minutes | **Serves:** 3

Per Serving: Calories 210 | Total Fat 3g | Protein 8g | Carbs 13g | Fiber: 2g

Ingredients:

- 1 teaspoon of olive oil
- 2 medium salmon fillets, boneless
- 1 teaspoon of sweet paprika
- A pinch of salt and black pepper
- 1 teaspoon of lemon juice
- 1 garlic clove, minced

For the salsa:

- 1 cup of chopped red bell pepper
- ½ teaspoon of chopped oregano
- 1 small habanero pepper, chopped
- ¼ cup of chopped green onions
- 1 garlic clove, minced
- ¼ cup of lemon juice

Directions:

- Combine red bell pepper, salt, habanero, 1/4 cup lemon juice, 1 garlic clove, green onion, oregano, and black pepper in a mixing bowl. In another large mixing bowl, combine paprika, 1 garlic clove, olive oil, and four teaspoons of lemon juice.
- Stir in the fish, then rub it with the spice mixture for 10 minutes. Season the fish using sea salt and black pepper and cook for 5 minutes on each side on a grill pan on medium-high flame. Divide among dishes, cover with salsa, and serve.
- Enjoy!

10. Salmon with Balsamic Fennel
Preparation time: 10 minutes | **Cooking time:** 20 minutes | **Serves:** 4

Per Serving: Calories 200 | Total Fat 2g | Protein 8g | Carbs 10g | Fiber: 4g

Ingredients:

- 1 tablespoon of balsamic vinegar

- 2 boneless salmon fillets
- 1 tablespoon of olive oil
- Salt and black pepper to taste
- 1 tablespoon of lime juice
- ½ teaspoon of cumin, ground
- 2 fennel bulbs, shredded
- ½ teaspoon of oregano, dried
- 1 tablespoon of chives, chopped

Directions:

- Heat the oil inside a pan on medium flame, then add the fennel and cook for 5 minutes, stirring occasionally.
- Sear the salmon for 2 minutes on every side.
- Cook for 10 minutes more after adding the rest of the ingredients, then divide across plates and serve.

11. Chicken Chili

Preparation time: 10 minutes | **Cooking time:** 60 minutes | **Serves:** 4

Per Serving: Calories 300 | Total Fat 2g | Protein 11g | Carbs 15g | Fiber: 10g

Ingredients:

- 2 cups of chicken stock
- 1 chopped yellow onion
- 1 garlic cloves, minced
- 1 tablespoon of cocoa powder
- 1 pound of chicken breast, boneless, skinless, and cubed
- 1 tablespoon of cilantro, chopped
- 1 chopped green bell pepper
- ½ tablespoon of chili powder
- 1 teaspoon of smoked paprika
- 1 cup of canned tomatoes, chopped
- A pinch of salt and black pepper
- 1 tablespoon of olive oil

Directions:

- Heat the oil inside a pot on medium flame, then add the onion and garlic and cook for 5 minutes.
- Brown the meat after adding it for around 5 minutes.
- Toss in the remaining ingredients and simmer for 40 minutes over medium flame.
- Serve the chili in individual dishes for lunch.

12. Vegetable Curry

Preparation time: 10 minutes | **Cooking time:** 20 minutes | **Serves:** 4

Per Serving: Calories 121 | Total Fat 11g | Protein 2g | Carbs 6g | Fiber: 9g

Ingredients:

- 1 teaspoon of minced garlic
- 1 tablespoon of coconut oil
- ½ cup of coconut milk
- 1 medium onion, chopped
- 1 teaspoon of minced ginger
- ½ teaspoon of pepper
- 2 cups of broccoli florets
- 1 tablespoon of garam masala
- 2 cups of fresh spinach leaves
- ½ teaspoon of salt

Directions:

- Heat a nonstick pot on a high flame for one minute.
- Heat the oil for 2 minutes.
- Sauté for a minute after adding the garlic and ginger. Add the onions and garam masala and sauté for another minute.
- Simmer for 10 minutes with the remaining ingredients, except the spinach leaves.
- Stir in the spinach leaves, then turn off the flame and cover the saucepan for 5 minutes.
- Serve and enjoy!

13. Sea Bass Baked with Tomatoes, Olives & Capers
Preparation time: 10 minutes | **Cooking time:** 15 minutes | **Serves:** 4

Per Serving: Calories 273 | Total Fat 12g | Protein 35g | Carbs 5g | Fiber: 9g

Ingredients:

- 2 tablespoons of capers, drained
- ½ cup of chicken broth
- 4 (5-ounce) of sea bass fillets
- 1 cup of canned diced tomatoes
- 2 cups of packed spinach
- ½ cup of Kalamata olives, pitted, chopped
- 2 tablespoons of extra-virgin olive oil
- 1 teaspoon of salt
- ¼ teaspoon of ground black pepper
- 1 small onion, diced

Directions:

- Preheat your oven at 375°F.
- In a baking dish, drizzle the olive oil. Turn the fish fillets in the dish to cover both sides with oil.
- Add the onion, chicken stock, salt, tomatoes, olives, spinach, capers, and pepper to the fish.
- Place the baking dish in the preheated oven and cover using aluminum foil. Bake for around 15 minutes in the oven. Serve hot.

14. Chicken Breast with Cherry Sauce
Preparation time: 10 minutes | **Cooking time:** 30 minutes | **Serves:** 4

Per Serving: Calories 379 | Total Fat 14g | Protein 43g | Carbs 17g | Fiber: 4g

Ingredients:
- 4 boneless & skinless chicken breasts
- ½ cup of dried cherries
- 1 tablespoon of coconut oil
- 2 scallions, sliced
- ¾ cup of chicken broth
- Salt & pepper to taste
- 1 tablespoon of balsamic vinegar

Directions:
- Preheat your oven at 375°F.
- Melt the coconut oil in an ovenproof skillet.
- Season the chicken well using salt and pepper. Brown it on both sides in the pan, approximately 3 minutes on each side.
- Add the scallions, balsamic vinegar, chicken broth, and cherries. Transfer the pan to the preheated oven. Cover and bake for 20 minutes. Serve hot.

15. Sauté Chicken and Bell Pepper
Preparation time: 10 minutes | **Cooking time:** 15 minutes | **Serves:** 4

Per Serving: Calories 179 | Total Fat 13g | Protein 10g | Carbs 6g | Fiber: 1g

Ingredients:
- 1 chopped red bell pepper
- 5 minced garlic cloves
- 1/4 teaspoon of ground black pepper
- 1 chopped onion
- 1 1/2 pounds of boneless and skinless chicken breasts, make bite-size chunks
- 3 tablespoons of extra-virgin olive oil
- 1/2 teaspoon of sea salt

Directions:
- Warm the olive oil in a large-sized nonstick skillet on medium-high flame till it shimmers.
- Add the onion, red bell pepper, and chicken. Cook, stirring periodically, for 10 minutes.
- Add the salt, garlic, and pepper to taste. Cook for 30 seconds while constantly stirring.

16. Roasted Salmon and Asparagus
Preparation time: 10 minutes | **Cooking time:** 15 minutes | **Serves:** 4

Per Serving: Calories 308 | Total Fat 18g | Protein 36g | Carbs 5g | Fiber: 2g

Ingredients:
- 1 pound of asparagus spears, trimmed

- 2 tablespoons of extra-virgin olive oil
- 1/4 teaspoon of ground black pepper
- 1 teaspoon of sea salt divided
- Zest and slices of 1 lemon
- 1 1/2 pounds of salmon, make four fillets

Directions:

- Preheat your oven at 425°F.
- Toss the asparagus with 1/2 teaspoon of salt and the olive oil. Spread evenly in the roasting pan.
- Season the fish with the remaining 1/2 teaspoon of salt and pepper. Place the asparagus on top, skin side down.
- Sprinkle the lemon zest over the salmon and asparagus, and garnish with the lemon slices.
- Bake for around 12 to 15 minutes in a preheated oven till the flesh is opaque.

17. Roasted Vegetables with Sweet Potatoes and White Beans
Preparation time: 15 minutes | **Cooking time:** 25 minutes | **Serves:** 4

Per Serving: Calories 315 | Total Fat 13g | Protein 10g | Carbs 32g | Fiber: 13g

Ingredients:

- 1 tablespoon of minced or grated lemon zest
- 1 teaspoon of salt
- 2 small dice sweet potatoes
- 1 medium peeled and thinly sliced carrot
- ¼ cup of extra-virgin olive oil
- ½ red onion, make ¼-inch dice
- 1 (15½-ounce) can of drained and rinsed white beans
- 4 ounces of green beans, trimmed
- 1 tablespoon of chopped fresh dill
- ¼ teaspoon of ground black pepper

Directions:

- Preheat your oven at 400°F.
- On a large-rimmed baking sheet, combine the green beans, sweet potatoes, salt, onion, carrot, oil, and pepper. Arrange everything in a single layer.
- Transfer to the oven.
- Roast for around 20 to 25 minutes or until the vegetables are soft.
- Mix in the lemon zest, white beans, and dill before serving.

18. Garlicky Chicken and Vegetables
Preparation time: 10 minutes | **Cooking time:** 45 minutes | **Serves:** 4

Per Serving: Calories 315 | Total Fat 8g | Protein 44g | Carbs 12g | Fiber: 2g

Ingredients:

- 1 leek, thinly sliced, white part only
- 4 bone-in, skin-on chicken breasts

- 2 teaspoons of extra-virgin olive oil
- Juice of 1 lemon
- 2 large zucchinis, make ¼-inch slices
- ½ cup of chicken broth
- 1 teaspoon of salt
- 3 minced garlic cloves
- 1 teaspoon of dried oregano
- ¼ teaspoon of ground black pepper

Directions:

- Preheat your oven at 400°F. Brush the baking sheet using oil.
- Place the zucchini and leeks on a baking sheet.
- Sprinkle the garlic, oregano, salt, and pepper over the chicken, skin-side up. Pour in the chicken stock.
- Transfer to the oven.
- Cook for around 35 to 40 minutes. Remove and set aside for 5 minutes to rest.
- Serve with the lemon juice.

19. Turkey Breast with Golden Vegetables
Preparation time: 10 minutes | **Cooking time:** 45 minutes | **Serves:** 4

Per Serving: Calories 383 | Total Fat 15g | Protein 37g | Carbs 25g | Fiber: 3g

Ingredients:

- ½ boneless and skin-on turkey breast (1 to 2 pounds)
- 1 teaspoon of turmeric
- 2 large golden beets, peeled and thinly sliced
- ½ medium yellow onion, thinly sliced
- 2 tablespoons of honey
- 1 teaspoon of salt
- 1 medium acorn squash, seeded and thinly sliced
- ¼ teaspoon of ground black pepper
- 2 tablespoons of olive oil
- 1 cup of chicken broth or vegetable broth

Directions:

- Preheat your oven at 400°F. Using the oil, grease a baking sheet.
- Arrange the beets, squash, and onion on a baking pan in a single layer. Place the turkey skin-side up on a plate. Drizzle the honey over the top.
- Add the broth and season using salt, turmeric, and pepper.
- Roast for around 35 to 45 minutes or until an instant-read thermometer reads 165°F in the middle of the turkey. Remove and set aside for 5 minutes to rest.
- Cut into slices and serve.

20. Tilapia with Asparagus and Acorn Squash

Preparation time: 10 minutes | **Cooking time:** 30 minutes | **Serves:** 4

Per Serving: Calories 246 | Total Fat 8g | Protein 25g | Carbs 17g | Fiber: 4g

Ingredients:

- 1-pound of asparagus, trim the woody ends and make 2-inch pieces
- 2 tablespoons of extra-virgin olive oil
- 1 tablespoon of chopped fresh flat-leaf parsley
- 1-pound of tilapia fillets
- 1 medium acorn squash, seeded and thinly sliced
- ¼ teaspoon of ground black pepper
- 1 large shallot, thinly sliced
- ½ cup of chicken broth
- 1 teaspoon of salt

Directions:

- Preheat your oven at 400°F. Brush the baking sheet with oil.
- Arrange the asparagus, squash, and shallot on a baking sheet in a single layer. Roast for 8 to 10 minutes.
- Arrange the tilapia and pour the chicken broth over it.
- Season using salt, parsley, and pepper.
- Roast for another 15 minutes. Remove and set aside for 5 minutes before serving.

Chapter 10: Side Dishes and Seasonings

1. Green Beans with Crispy Shallots
Preparation time: 10 minutes | **Cooking time:** 20 minutes | **Serves:** 4

Per Serving: Calories 146 | Total Fat 13g | Protein 2g | Carbs 9g | Fiber: 4g

Ingredients:

- 1 tablespoon of chopped fresh tarragon
- ¼ cup of extra-virgin olive oil
- 1 pound of green beans, trimmed
- 1 large shallot, sliced thin
- Freshly ground black pepper
- 1 teaspoon of sea salt, plus extra for seasoning

Directions:

- Over a high flame, bring a large saucepan of water to a boil.
- Add a single teaspoon of sea salt to the boiling water before adding the beans. Cook for 5 minutes or until they turn brilliant green.
- Transfer the beans to a serving plate after draining.
- Warm the olive oil in a small saucepan on medium flame. Add the shallots once the oil is heated. Cook for 1–2 minutes, till the edges begin to brown.
- Serve the shallots on top of the green beans. Season using sea salt and pepper and sprinkle with tarragon.

2. Rosemary Squash
Preparation time: 10 minutes | **Cooking time:** 40 minutes | **Serves:** 4

Per Serving: Calories 116 | Total Fat 5g | Protein 2g | Carbs 17g | Fiber: 2g

Ingredients:

- 2 sweet potatoes, unpeeled
- 2 winter squash, such as acorn or spaghetti
- ½ teaspoon of sea salt or to taste
- 3 tablespoons of extra-virgin olive oil
- ¼ teaspoon of pepper
- 2 teaspoons of rosemary

Directions:

- Remove the shell from the squash and seed it before chopping it into 3/4-inch cubes.
- Sweet potatoes should be cut into 3/4-inch slices.
- Combine the sweet potatoes and squash, drizzle using olive oil, and season to taste.
- Bake for 40 minutes, covered. During the baking process, stirring occasionally.

3. Scrumptious Green Beans
Preparation time: 10 minutes | **Cooking time:** 30 minutes | **Serves:** 4

Per Serving: Calories 68 | Total Fat 5g | Protein 2g | Carbs 6g | Fiber: 2g

Ingredients:

- 1 pound of green beans, washed and trimmed
- 2 tablespoons of olive oil
- ¼ teaspoon of turmeric
- ½-inch cube of peeled ginger, julienned cut
- ½ teaspoon of ground cumin
- 1 teaspoon of sea salt
- ½ teaspoon of black or yellow mustard seeds
- 2 tablespoons of minced fresh cilantro
- ¼ cup of water
- Juice of 1 lemon

Directions:

- Over medium flame, sauté mustard seeds and ginger in olive oil till mustard seeds begin to burst.
- Stir in the beans for about 5 minutes over medium flame.
- Cover and simmer for 5 minutes after adding the water.
- When the majority of the water has evaporated, remove the cover. Cook till the beans are heated but still slightly crunchy, adding the additional ingredients except the lemon juice.
- Just before serving, squeeze in the lemon juice. Serve hot.

4. Simple & Delectable Beets
Preparation time: 10 minutes | **Cooking time:** 30 minutes | **Serves:** 4

Per Serving: Calories 26 | Total Fat 0.1g | Protein 1g | Carbs 6g | Fiber: 1g

Ingredients:

- 1 teaspoon of lemon juice
- 3 beets, peeled and steamed till tender but still slightly crunchy
- Sea salt and pepper to taste
- 1 teaspoon of honey (optional)

Directions:

- Steam the beets and leave them aside to cool somewhat.
- In a 2-quart saucepan, combine the lemon juice and honey over a low flame till completely combined.
- Remove from flame. Slice the beets and add them to the pan. Mix carefully.
- Season using sea salt and pepper to taste, and serve immediately.
- If you don't want to use honey, simply season the beets using sea salt, lemon juice, and pepper and serve.

5. Lemon Garlic Brussel Sprouts
Preparation time: 10 minutes | **Cooking time:** 25 minutes | **Serves:** 4

Per Serving: Calories 72 | Total Fat 7g | Protein 1g | Carbs 3g | Fiber: 1g

Ingredients:

- 1 large lemon, zest and juice

- 2 pounds of Brussels sprouts, halved
- 3 tablespoons of avocado oil
- Salt and pepper to taste
- 5 cloves of garlic, chopped

Directions:

- Heat the avocado oil inside a large skillet on medium-high flame.
- Sauté Brussels sprouts for about 20 minutes or till soft.
- Add the garlic, lemon zest, and juice.
- Season to taste using salt and pepper.

6. Herb Salad Seasoning Mix
Preparation time: 5 minutes | **Cooking time:** 0 minutes | **Serves:** 4

Per Serving: Calories 17 | Total Fat 1g | Protein 1.4g | Carbs 1g | Fiber: 1g

Ingredients:

- 2 teaspoons of dried marjoram
- ½ cup of low-fat parmesan powder
- 2 teaspoons of dried chives
- 2 teaspoons of dried basil
- ½ teaspoon of freshly ground black pepper
- 2 teaspoons of garlic powder
- 1 tablespoon of dried parsley flakes
- 2 teaspoons of onion powder
- 2 teaspoons of paprika

Directions:

- Mix Parmesan powder, onion powder, chives, basil, marjoram, garlic powder, paprika, parsley flakes, and pepper in a small-sized mixing bowl; toss well to blend. Keep inside the airtight container.

7. Poultry Seasoning Mix
Preparation time: 5 minutes | **Cooking time:** 0 minutes | **Serves:** 4

Per Serving: Calories 2 | Total Fat 0g | Protein 0g | Carbs 1g | Fiber: 1g

Ingredients:

- 1 ½ teaspoons of ground dried thyme
- ¾ teaspoon of ground dried rosemary
- 2 teaspoons of ground-dried sage
- ½ teaspoon of ground nutmeg
- 1 teaspoon of ground-dried marjoram
- ½ teaspoon of finely ground black pepper

Directions:

- Combine sage, rosemary, nutmeg, thyme, marjoram, and black pepper in a sealable container; store till ready to use.

8. Turmeric Cauliflower

Preparation time: 10 minutes | **Cooking time:** 30 minutes | **Serves:** 3

Per Serving: Calories 168 | Total Fat 14g | Protein 4g | Carbs 10g | Fiber: 4g

Ingredients:

- 3 tablespoons of olive oil
- 1 large cauliflower head
- Salt to taste
- 2 teaspoons of turmeric

Directions:

- Preheat your oven at 400°F.
- Mix the turmeric, salt, and olive oil into the cauliflower florets.
- Arrange all ingredients on a cookie sheet and spread them out so they don't touch.
- Bake for around 25 to 30 minutes.
- Serve & enjoy!

9. Broccoli-Sesame Stir-Fry

Preparation time: 10 minutes | **Cooking time:** 10 minutes | **Serves:** 4

Per Serving: Calories 134 | Total Fat 11g | Protein 4g | Carbs 9g | Fiber: 3g

Ingredients:

- 1 teaspoon of sesame oil
- 2 minced garlic cloves
- 1 tablespoon of grated fresh ginger
- 2 tablespoons of toasted sesame seeds
- 1/4 teaspoon of sea salt
- 4 cups of broccoli florets
- 2 tablespoons of extra-virgin olive oil

Directions:

- Warm the olive oil and sesame oil inside a large-sized nonstick skillet on medium-high flame till they shimmer.
- Add the ginger, broccoli, and salt. Cook, stirring frequently, for 5 to 7 minutes or till the broccoli begins to color.
- Mix in the garlic. Cook for 30 seconds while constantly stirring.
- Take the pan off the flame and whisk in the sesame seeds.

10. Citrus Spinach

Preparation time: 10 minutes | **Cooking time:** 10 minutes | **Serves:** 4

Per Serving: Calories 80 | Total Fat 7g | Protein 1g | Carbs 4g | Fiber: 1g

Ingredients:

- 4 cups of fresh baby spinach
- 1/2 teaspoon of sea salt
- Juice of 1/2 orange

- 2 tablespoons of extra-virgin olive oil
- 1/4 teaspoon of ground black pepper
- 2 minced garlic cloves
- Zest of 1/2 orange

Directions:

- Warm the olive oil in a large skillet on medium-high flame till it shimmers.
- Cook for 3 minutes, stirring regularly, after adding the spinach.
- Mix in the garlic. Cook for 30 seconds while constantly stirring.
- Mix in the orange juice, zest, salt, and pepper. Cook, stirring continually, for about 2 minutes or till all of the juice evaporates.

11. Lemon-Pepper Seasoning Mix

Preparation time: 10 minutes | **Cooking time:** 25 minutes | **Serves:** 4

Per Serving: Calories 11 | Total Fat 0.2g | Protein 0.4g | Carbs 4g | Fiber: 0.5g

Ingredients:

- 2 lemons
- ¼ teaspoon of onion flakes
- 2 tablespoons of multi-colored peppercorns
- ¼ teaspoon of dehydrated minced garlic

Directions:

- Preheat your oven at 200°F. Line a baking sheet using parchment paper.
- Lemons should be washed and dried before use. Remove the zest off both lemons using a vegetable peeler, being careful not to get any of the pith. Put the peels in a single layer on the lined baking sheet.
- Bake for 25 minutes in a preheated oven, up to the point the peels have curled and dried. Allow the lemon peels to cool for about 20 minutes inside the turned-off oven, propped open with a wooden spoon to allow moisture to escape. Remove the pan from the oven and allow it to cool completely before proceeding to the next step.
- Combine dried lemon peels and peppercorns in a food processor fitted with a blade. Blend until the mixture is coarse. Add the dried onion and garlic and blend till smooth and well combined.

12. Creole Seasoning Blend Mix

Preparation time: 10 minutes | **Cooking time:** 0 minutes | **Serves:** 4

Per Serving: Calories 16 | Total Fat 0.4g | Protein 0.7g | Carbs 4g | Fiber: 0.5g

Ingredients:

- 1 tablespoon of black pepper
- 5 tablespoons of paprika
- 2 tablespoons of onion powder
- 2 tablespoons of dried basil
- 1 tablespoon of cayenne pepper
- 2 tablespoons of dried oregano
- 1 tablespoon of dried thyme
- 2 tablespoons of garlic powder

- 1 tablespoon of white pepper

Directions:

- Inside a small-sized mixing bowl, combine onion powder, white pepper, basil, garlic powder, oregano, black pepper, thyme, cayenne pepper, and paprika. Keep the container tightly closed after adding the seasoning mix.

13. Garam Masala
Preparation time: 10 minutes | **Cooking time:** 0 minutes | **Serves:** 4

Per Serving: Calories 8 | Total Fat 0.2g | Protein 0.2g | Carbs 1g | Fiber: 0.4g

Ingredients:

- 1 teaspoon of ground cinnamon
- 1 ½ teaspoons of ground cardamom
- ½ teaspoon of ground clove
- 1 ½ teaspoons of ground black pepper
- 1 tablespoon of ground cumin
- 1 ½ teaspoons of ground coriander
- ½ teaspoon of ground nutmeg

Directions:

- Combine cumin, cinnamon, pepper, coriander, cloves, cardamom, and nutmeg inside a mixing bowl. Keep the mixture cool and dry in an airtight container.

14. Rosemary and Garlic Sweet Potatoes
Preparation time: 10 minutes | **Cooking time:** 20 minutes | **Serves:** 4

Per Serving: Calories 199 | Total Fat 7g | Protein 2g | Carbs 33g | Fiber: 5g

Ingredients:

- 2 sweet potatoes with skin on, make 1/2 inch cubes
- 3 minced garlic cloves
- 1 tablespoon of chopped rosemary leaves
- 1/2 teaspoon of ground black pepper
- 2 tablespoons of extra-virgin olive oil
- 1/2 teaspoon of sea salt

Directions:

- Warm the olive oil inside a large nonstick skillet over medium-high flame till it shimmers.
- Incorporate the rosemary, sweet potatoes, and salt. Cook, stirring periodically, for 10 to 15 minutes or till the sweet potatoes begin to brown.
- Mix in the garlic and pepper. Cook for 30 seconds while constantly stirring.

15. Brown Rice with Bell Peppers
Preparation time: 10 minutes | **Cooking time:** 10 minutes | **Serves:** 4

Per Serving: Calories 266 | Total Fat 8g | Protein 5g | Carbs 44g | Fiber: 3g

Ingredients:

- 1 chopped onion

- 2 tablespoons of low-sodium soy sauce
- 1 red bell pepper, chopped
- 2 cups of cooked brown rice
- 1 green bell pepper, chopped
- 2 tablespoons of extra-virgin olive oil

Directions:

- Warm the olive oil inside a large-sized nonstick skillet on medium-high flame till it shimmers.
- Add the red and green bell peppers, as well as the onion. Cook, stirring regularly, for about 7 minutes or till the veggies begin to brown.
- Mix in the rice and soy sauce. Cook for 3 minutes, stirring regularly, till the rice is heated.

Chapter 11: Sweets and Desserts

1. Green Tea–Poached Pears
Preparation time: 10 minutes | **Cooking time:** 15 minutes | **Serves:** 4

Per Serving: Calories 190 | Total Fat 1g | Protein 1g | Carbs 50g | Fiber: 7g

Ingredients:

- 1/4 cup of honey
- 4 pears, peeled, cored and quartered lengthwise
- 1 tablespoon of grated fresh ginger
- 2 cups of strongly brewed green tea

Directions:

- Combine the pears, honey, tea, and ginger inside a large-sized pot over medium-high flame. Bring to boil. Reduce the flame to medium-low, cover, and let the pears soften for about 15 minutes. Serve the pears with a spoonful of the poaching liquid on top.

2. Cranberry Compote
Preparation time: 5 minutes | **Cooking time:** 15 minutes | **Serves:** 4

Per Serving: Calories 172 | Total Fat 1g | Protein 1g | Carbs 39g | Fiber: 6g

Ingredients:

- Juice of 2 oranges
- 4 cups of fresh cranberries
- 1/4 cup of honey
- Zest of 1 orange
- 1 tablespoon of grated fresh ginger

Directions:

- Stir together the ginger, cranberries, orange juice, honey, and orange zest in a large pot on a medium-high flame. Bring the water to boil. Cook, stirring periodically, for approximately 10 minutes or till the cranberries pop and form a sauce. Refrigerate or serve immediately.

3. Cocoa Bites
Preparation time: 10 minutes | **Cooking time:** 0 minutes | **Serves:** 4

Per Serving: Calories 318 | Total Fat 33g | Protein 4g | Carbs 8g | Fiber: 3g

Ingredients:

- 2 cups of walnuts
- 1 tablespoon of coconut oil
- 8 dates, pitted and coarsely chopped
- 2/3 cup of raw cocoa powder
- 2 tablespoons of water
- 1 cup of shredded coconut

Directions:

- Inside a food processor or high-speed blender, combine all of the ingredients and blend till thoroughly blended. To bring the mixture together, add 1 teaspoon of water at a time.
- Take the mixture out of the blender and roll it into 1-inch balls.
- Refrigerate till firm, then serve.

4. Cocoa Pudding
Preparation time: 10 minutes | **Cooking time:** 0 minutes | **Serves:** 1

Per Serving: Calories 457 | Total Fat 11g | Protein 5g | Carbs 48g | Fiber: 12g

Ingredients:

- ¼ cup of pitted Medjool dates
- 1 tablespoon of raw cocoa powder
- ½ ripe avocado
- 1 medium, super-ripe banana
- ¼ cup of filtered water
- 2 tablespoons of raw honey

Directions:

- Blend all of the ingredients inside a high-speed blender till completely smooth. If the consistency has to be smoothed out, add a teaspoon of water at a time.
- Top with strawberries, walnuts, or raw cocoa nibs and serve in glass cups or tiny dessert dishes.

5. No Bake Carrot Cake Bites
Preparation time: 15 minutes | **Cooking time:** 0 minutes | **Serves:** 4

Per Serving: Calories 231 | Total Fat 12g | Protein 3g | Carbs 32g | Fiber: 5g

Ingredients:

- 1 tablespoon of pure maple syrup
- 1 ½ cups of carrots
- 1 cup of pitted Medjool dates
- ½ teaspoon of ground ginger
- 1 teaspoon of cinnamon
- ¾ cup of shredded coconut
- 1 cup of walnuts

Directions:

- Inside a high-speed blender or food processor, combine all of the ingredients and blend till smooth, incorporating a teaspoon of water at a time as necessary.
- Place the carrot mixture in a cupcake tray and press it down and chill till hard.
- Remove the carrot cakes from the muffin tray and serve!

6. Chocolate-Cherry Clusters
Preparation time: 15 minutes | **Cooking time:** 0 minutes | **Serves:** 4

Per Serving: Calories 198 | Total Fat 13g | Protein 4g | Carbs 18g | Fiber: 4g

Ingredients:

- 1 cup of roasted salted almonds

- 1 tablespoon of coconut oil
- ½ cup of dried cherries
- 1 cup of dark chocolate (60 percent cocoa or higher), chopped

Directions:

- Wax paper should be used to line a rimmed baking pan.
- Stir the chocolate and coconut oil together in a double boiler till melted and smooth.
- Remove from the flame and add the cherries and almonds.
- Drop clusters onto wax paper by spoonfuls. Refrigerate till firm.
- Place in an airtight jar and chill.

7. Chocolate-Avocado Mousse with Sea Salt
Preparation time: 10 minutes | **Cooking time:** 5 minutes | **Serves:** 4

Per Serving: Calories 653 | Total Fat 47g | Protein 7g | Carbs 56g | Fiber: 9g

Ingredients:

- 2 ripe avocados
- 8 ounces of bittersweet chocolate, chopped
- Pinch sea salt
- ¼ cup of coconut milk
- 2 tablespoons of coconut oil
- ¼ cup of raw honey or maple syrup

Directions:

- Combine the coconut milk, chocolate, and coconut oil in a small-sized heavy saucepan on low flame. Cook, stirring regularly, for 2 to 3 minutes or till the chocolate melts.
- Combine the avocado and honey in a food processor. Process the melting chocolate till smooth.
- Spoon the mousse into the bowls for serving and sprinkle with sea salt. Allow at least 30 minutes to chill before serving.

8. Blueberry Crisp
Preparation time: 10 minutes | **Cooking time:** 20 minutes | **Serves:** 4

Per Serving: Calories 497 | Total Fat 33g | Protein 5g | Carbs 51g | Fiber: 7g

Ingredients:

- 2 teaspoons of lemon zest
- ½ cup of coconut oil melted, plus extra for brushing
- 1 quart of fresh blueberries
- Juice of ½ lemon
- ½ teaspoon of ground cinnamon
- 1 cup of gluten-free rolled oats
- ½ cup of chopped pecans
- Pinch salt
- ¼ cup of maple syrup

Directions:

- Preheat your oven at 350°F.
- Melted coconut oil should be brushed over a shallow baking dish. In the dish, combine the blueberries, lemon juice, maple syrup, and lemon zest.
- In a small-sized mixing dish, combine the oats, 1/2 cup of melted coconut oil, pecans, cinnamon, and salt. To distribute the coconut oil evenly, thoroughly combine the ingredients. Sprinkle the oat mixture over the fruit.
- Bake for around 20 minutes, or till the oats are gently toasted, in a preheated oven.

9. Apricot Squares
Preparation time: 10 minutes | **Cooking time:** 0 minutes | **Serves:** 4

Per Serving: Calories 201 | Total Fat 15g | Protein 3g | Carbs 17g | Fiber: 2g

Ingredients:
- 1 cup of macadamia nuts, chopped
- 1 cup of apricot, chopped
- 1 cup of shredded coconut, dried
- 1 teaspoon of vanilla extract
- 1/3 cup of turmeric powder
- 1 cup of apricot, dried

Directions:
- Combine all of the ingredients inside a food processor.
- Pulse till the mixture is absolutely smooth.
- Fill a square pan midway with the ingredients and evenly press them together.
- After chilling, enjoy!

10. Chocolate Cherry Chia Pudding
Preparation time: 15 minutes | **Cooking time:** 0 minutes | **Serves:** 4

Per Serving: Calories 404 | Total Fat 16g | Protein 6g | Carbs 12g | Fiber: 3g

Ingredients:
- ½ tablespoon of raw cacao powder
- 1 tablespoon of maple syrup or honey
- ½ cup of sliced pitted cherries
- 1 1/2 cups of coconut or almond milk
- ¼ cup of chia seeds; you can also use chia seed powder
- 1 raw cacao nibs

Extra toppings:
- Dark chocolate shavings (Preferably 70% dark chocolate or more)
- Extra cherries

Directions:
- Make use of a bowl or a mason jar. In a mixing bowl, combine the maple syrup, milk, chia seeds or powder, and raw cacao. After thoroughly stirring, place in the refrigerator for at least 4 hours.
- If you prefer to use a mason jar, simply combine all of the ingredients in the jar, screw on the lid, and shake!

- Serve in separate dishes with any or all of the above toppings.
- Enjoy!

11. Dark Chocolate Granola Bars
Preparation time: 15 minutes | **Cooking time:** 25 minutes | **Serves:** 4

Per Serving: Calories 364 | Total Fat 20g | Protein 6g | Carbs 37g | Fiber: 4g

Ingredients:

- 2/3 cup of honey
- ¼ cup of dark cocoa powder
- 1 teaspoon of vanilla
- ¼ cup of flaxseeds
- 1 cup of walnuts
- ½ cup of dark chocolate chips
- 1 cup of tart cherries, dried
- 3 eggs
- 1 teaspoon of salt
- ½ cup of buckwheat

Directions:

- Preheat your oven at 350°F.
- Coat a baking sheet using cooking spray.
- In a food processor, combine the walnuts, wheat, salt, tart cherries, and flaxseed. Everything must be finely chopped.
- In a container, combine the honey, vanilla extract, eggs, and cocoa powder.
- Fill your container halfway with the wheat mixture. Blend thoroughly.
- Add the chocolate chips. Re-stir the mixture.
- Place this mixture in a baking dish.
- Drizzle chocolate chips and tart cherries over the top.
- Bake for approximately 25 minutes. Allow to cool before serving.

12. Blueberry Energy Bites
Preparation time: 10 minutes | **Cooking time:** 0 minutes | **Serves:** 4

Per Serving: Calories 93 | Total Fat 1g | Protein 3g | Carbs 13g | Fiber: 1g

Ingredients:

- ½ cup of unsweetened almond milk
- 2 tablespoons of dried blueberries
- ¼ teaspoon of cinnamon
- 2 tablespoons of pure maple syrup
- ½ cup of gluten-free oat flour
- 2 tablespoons of organic peanut butter
- ½ teaspoon of sea salt

Directions:

- Stir together the dry ingredients, including the peanut butter, in a mixing dish.
- Stir in the almond milk and maple syrup.
- Form into 1-inch balls and chill in the refrigerator before serving.

13. Coconut Butter Fudge
Preparation time: 10 minutes | **Cooking time:** 0 minutes | **Serves:** 4

Per Serving: Calories 334 | Total Fat 36g | Protein 0g | Carbs 6g | Fiber: 0g

Ingredients:
- 1 teaspoon of pure vanilla extract
- ¼ teaspoon of salt
- 1 tablespoon of raw honey
- 1 cup of coconut butter

Directions:
- To begin, line an 8x8-inch baking dish using parchment paper.
- Melt the honey, coconut butter, and vanilla in a small saucepan over low heat.
- Place the mixture in the baking pan and place it in the refrigerator for approximately 2 hours before serving.

14. Cookie Dough Bites
Preparation time: 10 minutes | **Cooking time:** 0 minutes | **Serves:** 4

Per Serving: Calories 373 | Total Fat 10g | Protein 13g | Carbs 59g | Fiber: 0g

Ingredients:
- 1 1/2 cups of chickpeas, cooked
- ¼ cup of almond flour
- ½ teaspoon of salt
- 1 teaspoon of vanilla extract
- ¼ cup of chocolate chips, dairy-free & sugar-free
- 1 tablespoon of maple syrup
- ½ cup of almond butter or any nut butter

Directions:
- First, in a high-speed blender, combine all of the ingredients except the chocolate chips for about 3 minutes or till you have a thick, creamy liquid.
- After that, transfer the mixture to a medium-sized container.
- After that, fold in the chocolate chunks.
- Check for sweetness and add additional maple syrup if necessary.
- Give the dough shape according to your likeness.
- Chill for some time and serve.

15. Raspberry Sorbet
Preparation time: 10 minutes | **Cooking time:** 0 minutes | **Serves:** 4

Per Serving: Calories 224 | Total Fat 16g | Protein 4g | Carbs 22g | Fiber: 1g

Ingredients:

- 1 teaspoon of honey
- 14 ounces/400 g of frozen raspberry
- Mint
- 1/5 cup of almond milk

Directions:

- Blend the almond milk and raspberry till smooth, then place the mixture in the freezer for 40 minutes.
- When ready to serve, place them in ice cream bowls and garnish using mint.

Part 3: An Anti-Inflammatory Lifestyle

Insight into the Anti-Inflammatory Lifestyle

While a nutritious diet is important in lowering inflammation, living an anti-inflammatory lifestyle entails more than just eating well. It includes different parts of your daily routine as well as decisions that can have a substantial impact on your overall well-being. Beyond nutrition, here are some insights on the anti-inflammatory lifestyle:

Exercise on a Regular Basis

Regular physical activity not only helps to maintain a healthy weight, but it also has anti-inflammatory properties. Exercise increases endorphin production, decreases stress, and improves circulation, all of which can help lower inflammation levels in the body. Incorporate a variety of cardiovascular, strength, and flexibility workouts into your routine.

Stress Reduction

Inflammation in the body can be exacerbated by chronic stress. Stress-reduction approaches such as meditation, yoga, deep breathing exercises, and mindfulness practices can all help. Find relaxing and unwinding hobbies, and prioritize self-care to reduce the negative influence of stress on your body.

Sleeping Well

A good night's sleep is critical for general health and inflammation management. The body repairs and replenishes itself when sleeping, including lowering inflammation. To guarantee peaceful and rejuvenating sleep, establish a regular sleep routine, create a pleasant sleeping environment, and practice good sleep hygiene behaviors.

Keeping a Healthy Weight

Obesity can contribute to chronic inflammation. You may assist in minimizing inflammation in the body by keeping a healthy weight with a balanced diet and frequent exercise. Concentrate on feeding your body nutritious nutrients and finding pleasurable methods to keep active.

Relaxation and Mindfulness Techniques

Incorporate relaxation and mindfulness techniques into your regular routine. Meditation, deep breathing exercises, writing, and spending time in nature are all activities that can help promote relaxation, reduce stress, and support an anti-inflammatory lifestyle.

Toxin Reduction and Environmental Stressors

Reduce your exposure to environmental chemicals and stressors that might cause inflammation. This includes not smoking, decreasing pollution exposure, utilizing natural and non-toxic cleaning and personal care products, and maintaining a clean and orderly living space.

Developing Healthy Relationships

Emotional well-being requires positive social connections and supportive partnerships. Surround yourself with people who are encouraging and supportive, engage in meaningful conversations, and take part in activities that promote a sense of connection and belonging.

Remember that living an anti-inflammatory lifestyle is a comprehensive approach that entails incorporating a variety of behaviors and activities into your daily routine. You can support your body's natural ability to lower inflammation and improve your overall well-being by emphasizing self-care, controlling stress, remaining physically active, and creating a happy atmosphere.

Chapter 12: Physical Activity and Exercise

When it comes to health advantages, nothing compares to exercising. This makes it easier to maintain a healthy body weight and level of fitness. Regular exercise is vital for staying healthy and disease-free. According to new research, physical activity helps reduce muscular inflammation. Working out, according to researchers at Duke University's Center for Biomedical Engineering and Sciences, can minimize the harmful consequences of chronic inflammation on human muscle. The study's findings were published in the journal Science Advances, according to ANI.

It is Important to Exercise Consistently

Exercising is important for a variety of reasons. It can help with weight loss and keep you physically active, robust, and disease-free. Exercise can be readily incorporated into your everyday routine without spending hundreds of dollars on a gym membership.

Simply do your favorite form of exercise, such as walking, running, cycling, or jogging. Aerobics, Zumba, and dance.

Furthermore, there is a range of workouts that may be performed without the use of any particular equipment or facilities. Many effective workouts can be finished in as little as ten minutes, making them excellent for people who are short on time. To begin exercising, all you actually need is willpower, commitment, and self-control.

12.1 Benefits of Exercise for Reducing Inflammation

One of the many health benefits of regular exercise is a lower level of inflammation throughout the body. Although inflammation is a normal response to infection or damage, it has been linked to major illnesses such as diabetes, cancer, and heart disease over time. The following are some of the ways that exercise can help reduce inflammation:

12.1.1 Strengthens the Body's Natural Anti-Inflammatory Response

Exercising can increase the production of cytokines and adiponectin, two anti-inflammatory chemicals that aid the body's response to inflammation.

12.1.2 Improves Insulin Sensitivity

Regular exercise can improve insulin sensitivity, which can help reduce inflammation. Type 2 diabetes and metabolic syndrome are both inflammatory illnesses with one thing in common: insulin resistance.

12.1.3 Reduces Visceral Fat

Visceral fat, or belly fat, has been related to chronic inflammation. Regular exercise can help reduce visceral fat while also reducing inflammation.

12.1.4 Reduces the Levels of Inflammatory Markers

Exercise lowers blood levels of inflammatory indicators such as C-reactive protein (CRP).

12.1.5 Improves the Body's Defenses

Regular exercise, which improves the immune system, can help reduce inflammation. The immune system is mostly responsible for inflammation, and physical activity has been found to reduce this reaction.

12.1.6 Improves Immune Function

The immune system is critical in inflammation as well as the body's response to injury and infection. Regular exercise has been shown to boost the immune system's ability to manage inflammation and promote a more balanced immunological response.

12.1.7 Encourages Weight Management

Obesity and excess weight are closely connected to chronic inflammation. Physical activity helps with weight loss by burning calories, improving metabolism, and maintaining lean muscle mass. Maintaining a healthy weight reduces stress and inflammation in the body.

12.1.8 Improves Mental Health Conditions and Stress

Inflammation can be exacerbated by chronic stress and mental health issues. Exercise has been shown to lower stress and improve mood by increasing endorphin production, the body's natural feel-good hormones. Exercise indirectly reduces inflammation by lowering stress and boosting mental well-being.

Sticking to a regular exercise regimen is critical for reducing systemic inflammation and promoting health. To avoid damage, however, exercise should be started carefully and gradually increased in time and intensity. If you have a prior medical problem, you must consult with your doctor before beginning any new fitness plan.

12.2 Tips for Incorporating Physical Activity into Daily Life

Including physical activity in your regular routine is essential for reaping the advantages of exercise and lowering inflammation. Here are some helpful hints to help you incorporate physical activity into your daily routine:

12.2.1 Begin Slowly and Gradually Increase

Start with small, attainable goals if you're new to exercise or have a sedentary lifestyle. Begin with 10-15 minutes of movement daily and progressively increase the duration and intensity as time passes. This method will help you increase endurance and avoid injury.

12.2.2 Select Activities You Will Enjoy

Discover physical activities that you truly appreciate. Dancing, hiking, swimming, cycling, or even strolling are all possibilities. It's simpler to stay motivated and make exercise a habit when you enjoy it.

12.2.3 Set Attainable Objectives

Set goals that are reasonable and doable for your fitness level and schedule. Set a weekly goal of days or minutes of activity and track your progress. Celebrate your achievements and use them to motivate you to keep going.

12.2.4 Make it a Practice

Make physical activity a non-negotiable component of your day by incorporating it into your everyday routine. Schedule exercise time just as you would any other essential appointment or commitment.

12.2.5 Keep Moving Throughout the Day

Look for ways to be active throughout the day. If you work at a desk, take the stairs instead of the elevator, walk or cycle to local destinations instead of driving, and take brief breaks to stretch and move around.

12.2.6 Involve Family and Friends

Exercise with your friends, family, or coworkers. It not only improves the enjoyment of the exercise, but it also gives social support and accountability. Plan outdoor activities, join group exercise programs, or simply walk with your friends.

12.2.7 Make it Enjoyable

Try new hobbies, explore new places, or listen to music or podcasts while exercising to keep your exercises interesting and exciting. Adding variation and fun to your routine might help it become more pleasurable and sustainable.

12.2.8 Be Adaptable and Flexible

Because life can be unpredictable, keep your exercise program adaptable. Find alternate ways to be active if you miss a planned workout. Be willing to adapt your schedule or try new activities to accommodate changes in your everyday life.

12.3 What Workouts Can Help Reduce Inflammation?

One of the most significant things you can do for your health and way of life is to start exercising regularly. There are several ways in which regular exercise can improve your quality of life. Among individuals aged 40 and up, an estimated 110,000 deaths may be avoided annually if only more people engaged in regular physical activity. Among the many health benefits of exercise is a decrease in inflammatory risk factors.

12.3.1 Walking

Inflammation can be reduced with even light activities like walking. One of the easiest and most accessible ways to get some exercise is by going for a walk, which also happens to be one of the least expensive and most fun. A treadmill is a great way to get in some walking time whether you're at the gym or at home. Treadmills allow you to tailor your workout to your own level of effort and intensity. Instead, you may get started for very little money if you choose to stroll outside in nature. Walking outside in the fresh air has the added benefit of stimulating your senses by exposing you to the sights, sounds, and fragrances of nature.

12.3.2 Lifting Weights

Diseases associated with inflammation, such as obesity, coronary heart disease, and type 2 diabetes, can be mitigated with weight training. Gaining the advantages of resistance exercise does not require you to be a weightlifting prodigy. Working with weights can aid in both muscle growth and fat loss. Start with push-ups, squats, and pull-ups for some basic weight-resistance exercises. This easy weight-training routine helps you strengthen your upper and lower body and doesn't cost anything to get started. Joining a gym gives you access to a personal fitness instructor and exercise equipment you wouldn't have at home if you like weightlifting on your own. A personal trainer can help you lift weights in a secure manner if you are a beginner.

12.3.3 Yoga

Yoga is a great practice to incorporate into your workout routine if you're looking to calm your mind and body. Your state of mind can either stimulate or quell inflammation. Yoga can be done either alone or with others. Yoga incorporates both controlled breathing and slow, deliberate movements. Stress and anxiety can be reduced by yoga, making it easier to handle difficult situations.

12.3.4 Cycling

Riding a bike is the quickest and surest way to relive your glory days as a kid. To reap the benefits, a high-intensity spin class isn't necessary. Cycling has been shown to reduce inflammation, whether you choose to ride outdoors or on a stationary cycle.

Biking is a fantastic low-impact activity for those who suffer from joint pain or arthritis. In addition, riding increases hip and knee flexion and extension.

The goal is to develop a healthy lifestyle that includes frequent physical activity. Consistency is essential, so find ways to incorporate exercise into your daily routine that you actually love. Pay attention to your body, stay motivated, and enjoy your accomplishments along the road. With these methods, you may successfully include physical exercise into your routine and get the multiple benefits it provides in terms of inflammation reduction and overall health improvement.

Chapter 13: Stress Management and Emotional Well-Being

13.1 Connection Between Stress and Inflammation

The "fight-or-flight" response is our body's natural reaction to stress, and it helps us stay safe in dangerous situations. However, long-term stress has been linked to negative health outcomes, such as increased inflammation. In order to properly manage stress and inflammation, it is essential to understand the relationship between the two.

Stress causes the release of chemicals like cortisol and adrenaline, which set off a cascade of reactions in the body. These reactions can exacerbate inflammation by inhibiting anti-inflammatory, immune responses and promoting the generation of pro-inflammatory substances. Conditions including cardiovascular disease, immunological illnesses, and chronic pain can develop from this persistent, low-level inflammation.

Indirectly, stress can cause inflammation through the actions and decisions we make. When people are under a lot of pressure, they may resort to harmful coping techniques like binge eating, drinking too much, or smoking. All of these behaviors add to inflammation and worsen the body's health.

Also, stress might make it harder to fall asleep, digest food properly, and repair and regenerate damaged cells. Inflammation and the body's ability to heal normally can both be exacerbated by these disturbances.

Fortunately, there are ways to control stress and lessen its inflammatory effects. Mindfulness meditation, deep breathing exercises, regular physical activity, and hobbies or activities that induce relaxation are all effective stress management approaches.

In addition to stress management, other important factors in lowering inflammation due to stress include eating an anti-inflammatory diet, getting enough sleep, and making self-care a priority.

Individuals can take preventative measures to safeguard their health and well-being by learning to identify stressful situations, developing a plan to deal with them, and then putting that plan into action. Find healthy strategies to deal with stress if you want to keep your life in check and avoid inflammation.

13.2 Strategies for Reducing Stress and Improving Emotional Well-Being

There are many methods available for dealing with stress. To reap the greatest benefit, practice these methods often rather than only when stress symptoms arise. The majority of folks who seek relief do it through multiple channels.

13.2.1 Relaxation Techniques
Laugh more often

Laughter has been shown in studies to lower the stress hormone cortisol. It also improves your mood. Get together with someone who helps you laugh or watch a hilarious show.

Relax your mind

Mindfulness, massage, meditation, and deep breathing techniques can all help to reduce your heart rate and relax your mind. You can also enjoy relaxing sounds or your favorite music.

13.2.2 Physical Techniques
Engage in physical activity

Walking outside or working out with friends can help lift your spirits. You can also engage in mindful physical exercises such as yoga or tai chi.

Maintain a nutritious diet

Increase your intake of fresh vegetables and fruits. Reduce your intake of greasy meals, caffeine, and sugar.

Improve your sleeping patterns

To sleep better, turn off technology, establish a relaxing setting, and relax with a book or a warm bath.

Stop consuming substances

Quit smoking and limit your alcohol consumption.

13.2.3 Cognitive Techniques
Maintain a journal

Make a list of your accomplishments for the day. You can also record three positive events from the day or three things for which you are grateful.

Make "me time" a priority

Try to do a minimum of one thing for yourself every day. It could be meditating, socializing with a buddy, reading a book, or pursuing a pastime.

Seek assistance

A mental health expert can assist you in learning better stress management skills. Cognitive behavioral therapy (CBT) is a tried-and-true strategy for changing how you react to life's stresses.

Express your emotions

Connect with a trustworthy loved one or friend when you are feeling overwhelmed. Hearing a voice, whether in person or over the phone, can be beneficial.

Take command

To better organize your time and reduce to-dos, use lists or smartphone apps. Plan your day the night before so you know what you can anticipate — and what you may need to postpone. Allow yourself to decline other people's requests.

Everyone's path to stress reduction and emotional well-being is unique. Investigate many tactics to see which one works best for you. You may foster resilience, reduce stress, and improve your overall emotional well-being by emphasizing self-care and implementing good coping techniques.

Chapter 14: Sleep and Rest

14.1 Importance of Sleep in Reducing Inflammation

Sleep is an essential component of our general health and well-being, and its significance in inflammation reduction should not be overlooked. Adequate and restorative sleep is critical for maintaining a balanced immune system and fostering optimal physical function. Chronic sleep deprivation or poor-quality sleep, on the other hand, might contribute to increased inflammation in the body.

During sleep, our bodies undergo important vital processes such as hormone regulation, tissue repair, and immune system modulation. Inadequate sleep disturbs these mechanisms, resulting in an imbalance in our bodies inflammatory response. Sleep deprivation has been found in studies to increase the production of pro-inflammatory cytokines, or chemicals that promote inflammation while decreasing the production of anti-inflammatory cytokines.

Inadequate sleep can also hinder the body's capacity to regulate stress chemicals like cortisol, leading to increased stress and aggravating inflammation. Chronic sleep deprivation has been related to an increased risk of acquiring inflammatory diseases such as cardiovascular disease, diabetes, and autoimmune illnesses.

Improving sleep quality and length is critical for inflammation reduction and general health promotion. Appropriate sleep practices, also known as sleep hygiene, can help you achieve therapeutic and inflammation-reducing sleep. This involves creating a suitable sleep environment, practicing relaxation techniques before bedtime, and minimizing exposure to stimulating activities and technological gadgets in the evening.

Incorporating regular exercise into your daily routine will also help you sleep better and control your body's inflammatory response. Physical activity improves sleep and strengthens the body's inherent anti-inflammatory capabilities.

Sleep is an essential component of an anti-inflammatory lifestyle for reducing inflammation and sustaining good health. Adopting appropriate sleep habits and prioritizing sleep can help your body's natural healing processes, decrease inflammation, and improve overall well-being. Remember that a good night's sleep is a vital asset in your quest for a healthy, inflammation-free lifestyle.

14.2 Tips to Improve Sleep Quality and Promote Adequate Rest

If you have chronic inflammation and aren't receiving seven to nine hours of good sleep every night, you should consider how you might prioritize obtaining more sleep. While sleep disorders can be difficult to identify and even harder to treat, the following tips for modest lifestyle modifications can help you sleep better.

14.2.1 Maintain a Consistent Sleep Routine

Limit your sleep time to no more than eight hours. For optimal health, adults should get at least seven hours of sleep per night. Most people can function normally after sleeping for only eight hours.

Keep a regular schedule for sleeping and waking up, even on the weekends. Maintaining a regular schedule helps your body's circadian cycles.

If you're in bed for 20 minutes and still awake, you should go do something soothing. Relaxing music or calming reading material. If you're feeling sleepy, head back to bed. You can do this as often as necessary, but you should stick to the same bedtime and wake-up time each day.

14.2.2 Watch What You Put into Your Body

Avoid being very hungry or full before bed. In particular, don't have a big dinner less than two hours before bed. The inconvenience could keep you awake.

Caffeine, nicotine, and alcohol all need a word of warning. Nicotine and caffeine both have energizing effects that last for hours and might make it difficult to fall asleep. And while alcohol can produce drowsiness initially, it can cause sleep disruptions later on.

14.2.3 Make a Relaxing Environment

Always maintain a comfortable temperature, complete darkness, and silence in your bedroom. It may be more difficult to get to sleep if you're exposed to light in the evening. It's best to put away any screens that emit light several hours before night. You may use a fan, earplugs, and blackout curtains to create a comfortable atmosphere.

Better sleep may result from engaging in relaxing activities like taking a bath or practicing relaxation techniques right before bed.

14.2.4 Practice Meditation

The benefits of incorporating meditation into your daily routine are numerous. Research suggests that it may also help lower inflammation in the body, in addition to easing stress and facilitating restful sleep. Positive effects can be shown after even brief periods of practice, and there are many useful applications and websites to get you started.

14.2.5 Avoid Taking Long Naps During the Day

Interruption of nighttime sleep by long naps during the day is possible. Naps shouldn't last longer than an hour, and late-day naps should be avoided entirely.

Night shift workers, on the other hand, may need to catch up on sleep with a late-afternoon nap before heading into the office.

14.2.6 Do Some Sort of Physical Activity Every Day

Regular exercise may result in improved sleep. However, try to get some rest before going to bed.

Daily outdoor activities may also be useful.

14.2.7 Worry Less

Don't go to sleep worrying about things you can't control. Write down your thoughts and put them away for tomorrow.

Managing stress could be useful. Get back to fundamentals by establishing order, establishing priorities, and assigning responsibilities. Worry can also be reduced through meditation.

12 Weeks Meal Plan

Week 1

Day	Breakfast	Snack	Lunch	Snack	Dinner
1	Fruity Flaxseed Breakfast Bowl	Blueberry Crisp	Sweet Potato Curry with Spinach	Cocoa Pudding	Salmon with Salsa
2	Savory Breakfast Pancakes	Green Tea–Poached Pears	Chicken and Broccoli	No-Bake Golden Energy Bites	Eggplant and Tomato Stew
3	Blueberry Breakfast Blend	No Bake Carrot Cake Bites	Salmon with Balsamic Fennel	Zucchini Chips	Anti-Inflammatory Kale Salad
4	Breakfast Burgers with Avocado Buns	Golden Milk Chia Pudding	Moroccan Lentil Soup	Baked Kale Chips	Trout with Sweet-and-Sour Chard
5	Green Smoothie Bowl	Chocolate-Avocado Mousse with Sea Salt	Butternut Squash and Spinach Gratin with Lentils	Turmeric Nuggets	Braised Bok Choy with Shiitake Mushrooms
6	Breakfast Omelet	Cocoa Bites	Tilapia with Asparagus and Acorn Squash	Blueberry Crisp	Spinach Bean Salad
7	Kale Turmeric Scramble	Green Apple and Spinach Smoothie	Tuscany Vegetable Soup	Chocolate-Cherry Clusters	Turkey Breast with Golden Vegetables

Week 2

Day	Breakfast	Snack	Lunch	Snack	Dinner
1	Scrambled Eggs with Smoked Salmon	Smoked Turkey–Wrapped Zucchini Sticks	Garlicky Chicken and Vegetables	Kiwi Strawberry Smoothie	Buckwheat and Onion Soup
2	Breakfast Avocado Boat	Blueberry Smoothie	Roasted Vegetables with Sweet Potatoes and White Beans	Ginger Date Bars	Sea Bass Baked with Tomatoes, Olives & Capers
3	Herb Scramble with Sautéed Cherry Tomatoes	Cranberry Compote	Mediterranean Chopped Salad	Chocolate-Avocado Mousse with Sea Salt	Sauté Chicken and Bell Pepper

4	Green Smoothie Bowl	Cocoa Pudding	Coconut Fish Stew	Apricot Squares	Cabbage Orange Salad with Citrusy Vinaigrette
5	Breakfast Burgers with Avocado Buns	Dark Chocolate Granola Bars	Chicken Breast with Cherry Sauce	Green Tea–Poached Pears	Salmon Salad
6	Fruity Flaxseed Breakfast Bowl	Blueberry Energy Bites	Eggplant and Tomato Stew	Chocolate Cherry Chia Pudding	Tilapia with Asparagus and Acorn Squash
7	Breakfast Omelet	Coconut Butter Fudge	Roasted Salmon and Asparagus	Cookie Dough Bites	Roasted Vegetables with Sweet Potatoes and White Beans

Week 3

Day	Breakfast	Snack	Lunch	Snack	Dinner
1	Scrambled Eggs with Smoked Salmon	Zucchini Chips	Tomato Asparagus Frittata	Cranberry Compote	Sweet Potato Curry with Spinach
2	Blueberry Breakfast Blend	Roasted Cashews	Salmon with Salsa	Cocoa Bites	Sweet Potato Quinoa
3	Savory Breakfast Pancakes	Quinoa & Spinach Egg Bites	Spinach Bean Salad	Smoked Trout & Mango Wraps	Garlicky Chicken and Vegetables
4	Kale Turmeric Scramble	Coconut & Banana Cookies	Anti-Inflammatory Kale Salad	Fruity Bowl	Salmon with Balsamic Fennel
5	Breakfast Burgers with Avocado Buns	Raspberry Sorbet	Brown Rice with Bell Peppers	Apple Bruschetta with Almonds and Blackberries	Butternut Squash and Spinach Gratin with Lentils
6	Breakfast Burgers with Avocado Buns	Chocolate Cherry Chia Pudding	Buckwheat and Onion Soup	No Bake Carrot Cake Bites	Chicken Breast with Cherry Sauce
7	Blueberry Breakfast Blend	Pineapple Sticks	White Bean & Tuna Salad	Roasted Cashews	Roasted Salmon and Asparagus

Week 4

Day	Breakfast	Snack	Lunch	Snack	Dinner
1	Breakfast Omelet	Apricot Squares	Sauté Chicken and Bell Pepper	Blueberry Smoothie	Sea Bass Baked with Tomatoes, Olives & Capers
2	Herb Scramble with Sautéed Cherry Tomatoes	Cookie Dough Bites	Turkey Breast with Golden Vegetables	Green Apple and Spinach Smoothie	Mediterranean Chopped Salad
3	Fruity Flaxseed Breakfast Bowl	No-Bake Golden Energy Bites	Cabbage Orange Salad with Citrusy Vinaigrette	Green Tea and Pear Smoothie	Coconut Fish Stew
4	Kale Turmeric Scramble	Chocolate-Cherry Clusters	Chicken Breast with Cherry Sauce	Dark Chocolate Granola Bars	Chicken Chili
5	Breakfast Avocado Boat	Quinoa & Seeds Crackers	Garlicky Chicken and Vegetables	Coconut Butter Fudge	Moroccan Lentil Soup
6	Green Smoothie Bowl	Blueberry Crisp	Vegetable Curry	Smoked Turkey–Wrapped Zucchini Sticks	Chicken and Broccoli
7	Scrambled Eggs with Smoked Salmon	Baked Kale Chips	Sweet Potato Quinoa	Chocolate-Cherry Clusters	Tuscany Vegetable Soup

Week 5

Day	Breakfast	Snack	Lunch	Snack	Dinner
1	Fruity Flaxseed Breakfast Bowl	Blueberry Crisp	Sweet Potato Curry with Spinach	Cocoa Pudding	Salmon with Salsa
2	Savory Breakfast Pancakes	Green Tea–Poached Pears	Chicken and Broccoli	No-Bake Golden Energy Bites	Eggplant and Tomato Stew
3	Blueberry Breakfast Blend	No Bake Carrot Cake Bites	Salmon with Balsamic Fennel	Zucchini Chips	Anti-Inflammatory Kale Salad
4	Breakfast Burgers with Avocado Buns	Golden Milk Chia Pudding	Moroccan Lentil Soup	Baked Kale Chips	Trout with Sweet-and-Sour Chard

5	Green Smoothie Bowl	Chocolate-Avocado Mousse with Sea Salt	Butternut Squash and Spinach Gratin with Lentils	Turmeric Nuggets	Braised Bok Choy with Shiitake Mushrooms
6	Breakfast Omelet	Cocoa Bites	Tilapia with Asparagus and Acorn Squash	Blueberry Crisp	Spinach Bean Salad
7	Kale Turmeric Scramble	Green Apple and Spinach Smoothie	Tuscany Vegetable Soup	Chocolate-Cherry Clusters	Turkey Breast with Golden Vegetables

Week 6

Day	Breakfast	Snack	Lunch	Snack	Dinner
1	Herb Scramble with Sautéed Cherry Tomatoes	Cranberry Compote	Mediterranean Chopped Salad	Chocolate-Avocado Mousse with Sea Salt	Sauté Chicken and Bell Pepper
2	Green Smoothie Bowl	Cocoa Pudding	Coconut Fish Stew	Apricot Squares	Cabbage Orange Salad with Citrusy Vinaigrette
3	Breakfast Burgers with Avocado Buns	Dark Chocolate Granola Bars	Chicken Breast with Cherry Sauce	Green Tea–Poached Pears	Salmon Salad
4	Fruity Flaxseed Breakfast Bowl	Blueberry Energy Bites	Eggplant and Tomato Stew	Chocolate Cherry Chia Pudding	Tilapia with Asparagus and Acorn Squash
5	Breakfast Omelet	Coconut Butter Fudge	Roasted Salmon and Asparagus	Cookie Dough Bites	Roasted Vegetables with Sweet Potatoes and White Beans
6	Scrambled Eggs with Smoked Salmon	Zucchini Chips	Tomato Asparagus Frittata	Cranberry Compote	Sweet Potato Curry with Spinach
7	Blueberry Breakfast Blend	Roasted Cashews	Salmon with Salsa	Cocoa Bites	Sweet Potato Quinoa

Week 7

Day	Breakfast	Snack	Lunch	Snack	Dinner
1	Kale Turmeric Scramble	Coconut & Banana Cookies	Anti-Inflammatory Kale Salad	Fruity Bowl	Salmon with Balsamic Fennel
2	Breakfast Burgers with Avocado Buns	Raspberry Sorbet	Brown Rice with Bell Peppers	Apple Bruschetta with Almonds and Blackberries	Butternut Squash and Spinach Gratin with Lentils
3	Breakfast Burgers with Avocado Buns	Chocolate Cherry Chia Pudding	Buckwheat and Onion Soup	No Bake Carrot Cake Bites	Chicken Breast with Cherry Sauce
4	Blueberry Breakfast Blend	Pineapple Sticks	White Bean & Tuna Salad	Roasted Cashews	Roasted Salmon and Asparagus
5	Breakfast Omelet	Apricot Squares	Sauté Chicken and Bell Pepper	Blueberry Smoothie	Sea Bass Baked with Tomatoes, Olives & Capers
6	Herb Scramble with Sautéed Cherry Tomatoes	Cookie Dough Bites	Turkey Breast with Golden Vegetables	Green Apple and Spinach Smoothie	Mediterranean Chopped Salad
7	Fruity Flaxseed Breakfast Bowl	No-Bake Golden Energy Bites	Cabbage Orange Salad with Citrusy Vinaigrette	Green Tea and Pear Smoothie	Coconut Fish Stew

Week 8

Day	Breakfast	Snack	Lunch	Snack	Dinner
1	Breakfast Avocado Boat	Blueberry Smoothie	Roasted Vegetables with Sweet Potatoes and White Beans	Ginger Date Bars	Sea Bass Baked with Tomatoes, Olives & Capers
2	Herb Scramble with Sautéed Cherry Tomatoes	Cranberry Compote	Mediterranean Chopped Salad	Chocolate-Avocado Mousse with Sea Salt	Sauté Chicken and Bell Pepper
3	Green Smoothie Bowl	Cocoa Pudding	Coconut Fish Stew	Apricot Squares	Cabbage Orange Salad with Citrusy Vinaigrette
4	Breakfast Burgers with Avocado Buns	Dark Chocolate Granola Bars	Chicken Breast with Cherry Sauce	Green Tea–Poached Pears	Salmon Salad

5	Fruity Flaxseed Breakfast Bowl	Blueberry Energy Bites	Eggplant and Tomato Stew	Chocolate Cherry Chia Pudding	Tilapia with Asparagus and Acorn Squash
6	Breakfast Omelet	Coconut Butter Fudge	Roasted Salmon and Asparagus	Cookie Dough Bites	Roasted Vegetables with Sweet Potatoes and White Beans
7	Scrambled Eggs with Smoked Salmon	Zucchini Chips	Tomato Asparagus Frittata	Cranberry Compote	Sweet Potato Curry with Spinach

Week 9

Day	Breakfast	Snack	Lunch	Snack	Dinner
1	Blueberry Breakfast Blend	No Bake Carrot Cake Bites	Salmon with Balsamic Fennel	Zucchini Chips	Anti-Inflammatory Kale Salad
2	Breakfast Burgers with Avocado Buns	Golden Milk Chia Pudding	Moroccan Lentil Soup	Baked Kale Chips	Trout with Sweet-and-Sour Chard
3	Green Smoothie Bowl	Chocolate-Avocado Mousse with Sea Salt	Butternut Squash and Spinach Gratin with Lentils	Turmeric Nuggets	Braised Bok Choy with Shiitake Mushrooms
4	Breakfast Omelet	Cocoa Bites	Tilapia with Asparagus and Acorn Squash	Blueberry Crisp	Spinach Bean Salad
5	Kale Turmeric Scramble	Green Apple and Spinach Smoothie	Tuscany Vegetable Soup	Chocolate-Cherry Clusters	Turkey Breast with Golden Vegetables
6	Scrambled Eggs with Smoked Salmon	Smoked Turkey–Wrapped Zucchini Sticks	Garlicky Chicken and Vegetables	Kiwi Strawberry Smoothie	Buckwheat and Onion Soup
7	Breakfast Avocado Boat	Blueberry Smoothie	Roasted Vegetables with Sweet Potatoes and White Beans	Ginger Date Bars	Sea Bass Baked with Tomatoes, Olives & Capers

Week 10

Day	Breakfast	Snack	Lunch	Snack	Dinner
1	Scrambled Eggs with Smoked Salmon	Smoked Turkey–Wrapped Zucchini Sticks	Garlicky Chicken and Vegetables	Kiwi Strawberry Smoothie	Buckwheat and Onion Soup
2	Breakfast Avocado Boat	Blueberry Smoothie	Roasted Vegetables with Sweet Potatoes and White Beans	Ginger Date Bars	Sea Bass Baked with Tomatoes, Olives & Capers
3j	Herb Scramble with Sautéed Cherry Tomatoes	Cranberry Compote	Mediterranean Chopped Salad	Chocolate-Avocado Mousse with Sea Salt	Sauté Chicken and Bell Pepper
4	Green Smoothie Bowl	Cocoa Pudding	Coconut Fish Stew	Apricot Squares	Cabbage Orange Salad with Citrusy Vinaigrette
5	Breakfast Burgers with Avocado Buns	Dark Chocolate Granola Bars	Chicken Breast with Cherry Sauce	Green Tea–Poached Pears	Salmon Salad
6	Fruity Flaxseed Breakfast Bowl	Blueberry Energy Bites	Eggplant and Tomato Stew	Chocolate Cherry Chia Pudding	Tilapia with Asparagus and Acorn Squash
7	Breakfast Omelet	Coconut Butter Fudge	Roasted Salmon and Asparagus	Cookie Dough Bites	Roasted Vegetables with Sweet Potatoes and White Beans

Week 11

Day	Breakfast	Snack	Lunch	Snack	Dinner
1	Fruity Flaxseed Breakfast Bowl	Blueberry Crisp	Sweet Potato Curry with Spinach	Cocoa Pudding	Salmon with Salsa
2	Savory Breakfast Pancakes	Green Tea–Poached Pears	Chicken and Broccoli	No-Bake Golden Energy Bites	Eggplant and Tomato Stew
3	Blueberry Breakfast Blend	No Bake Carrot Cake Bites	Salmon with Balsamic Fennel	Zucchini Chips	Anti-Inflammatory Kale Salad

4	Breakfast Burgers with Avocado Buns	Golden Milk Chia Pudding	Moroccan Lentil Soup	Baked Kale Chips	Trout with Sweet-and-Sour Chard
5	Green Smoothie Bowl	Chocolate-Avocado Mousse with Sea Salt	Butternut Squash and Spinach Gratin with Lentils	Turmeric Nuggets	Braised Bok Choy with Shiitake Mushrooms
6	Breakfast Omelet	Cocoa Bites	Tilapia with Asparagus and Acorn Squash	Blueberry Crisp	Spinach Bean Salad
7	Kale Turmeric Scramble	Green Apple and Spinach Smoothie	Tuscany Vegetable Soup	Chocolate-Cherry Clusters	Turkey Breast with Golden Vegetables

Week 12

Day	Breakfast	Snack	Lunch	Snack	Dinner
1	Breakfast Omelet	Apricot Squares	Sauté Chicken and Bell Pepper	Blueberry Smoothie	Sea Bass Baked with Tomatoes, Olives & Capers
2	Herb Scramble with Sautéed Cherry Tomatoes	Cookie Dough Bites	Turkey Breast with Golden Vegetables	Green Apple and Spinach Smoothie	Mediterranean Chopped Salad
3	Fruity Flaxseed Breakfast Bowl	No-Bake Golden Energy Bites	Cabbage Orange Salad with Citrusy Vinaigrette	Green Tea and Pear Smoothie	Coconut Fish Stew
4	Kale Turmeric Scramble	Chocolate-Cherry Clusters	Chicken Breast with Cherry Sauce	Dark Chocolate Granola Bars	Chicken Chili
5	Breakfast Avocado Boat	Quinoa & Seeds Crackers	Garlicky Chicken and Vegetables	Coconut Butter Fudge	Moroccan Lentil Soup
6	Green Smoothie Bowl	Blueberry Crisp	Vegetable Curry	Smoked Turkey–Wrapped Zucchini Sticks	Chicken and Broccoli
7	Scrambled Eggs with Smoked Salmon	Baked Kale Chips	Sweet Potato Quinoa	Chocolate-Cherry Clusters	Tuscany Vegetable Soup

Shopping List

A

Almond flour
Avocado
Almond milk
Almond butter
Almond meal
Arugula
Almonds
Apple
Apple cider vinegar
Almond yogurt
Asparagus
Acorn squash
Avocado oil
Apricots

B

Berry
Bananas
Basil
Bell pepper
Blueberries
Black pepper
Broccoli
Blackberries
Balsamic vinegar
Black beans
Buckwheat
Brown rice
Bok choy
Butternut squash
Beets
Brussels Sprouts
Buckwheat

C

Cinnamon
Cranberries
Coconut flour
Coconut milk
Coconut yogurt
Coconut chips
Chia seeds
Chili powder
Cilantro
Chives
Cayenne pepper
Coconut oil
Coconut flakes
Cauliflower
Carrots
Cherry tomatoes
Cumin
Cashews
Chili flakes
Cherries
Coconut water
Cucumber
Chicken stock
Chickpeas
Celery
Cremini mushrooms
Cod fillets
Chervil
Clove
Chicken breasts
Chard
Curry powder
Coconut aminos
Cocoa powder
Capers
Cacao nibs
Coconut butter

D

Dates
Dijon mustard
Dried cherries
Dill

Dark chocolate

Dark cocoa powder

Dark chocolate chips

E

Eggs

Eggplant

F

Flaxseeds

Flaxseed meal

Fennel bulb

Filtered water

G

Ginger

Ground black pepper

Garlic

Green onions

Green tea

Garbanzo beans

Green cabbage

Garlic powder

Grapefruit

Golden raisins

Garam masala

Green beans

Golden beets

Ground cardamom

Ground clove

Ground coriander

Ground cumin

Ground black pepper

Ground nutmeg

Ground cinnamon

H

Honey

Herb seasoning

Hemp seeds

Hazelnuts

Habanero pepper

K

Kiwi

Kalamata olives

Kale

L

Lettuce leaf

Lemon

Lemon juice

Lime

Lemongrass

Lentils

Leek

Low-sodium soy sauce

M

Mushrooms

Maple syrup

Maca powder

Mango

Mint

Mustard seeds

Marjoram

Medjool dates

Macadamia nuts

N

Nutmeg

O

Olive oil

Oregano

Orange juice

Orange zest

Orange

Onion

Onion powder

Oat flour

Organic peanut butter

P

Protein powder

Parsley

Pineapple

Pears

Pineapple juice
Paprika
Parmesan powder
Peppercorns
Pecans

Q
Quinoa
Quinoa flour

R
Red onion
Raw sprouts
Raw honey
Red cabbage
Raspberry vinegar
Red lentils
Radishes
Raspberries
Rosemary
Raw cocoa powder
Rolled oats

S
Salt
Salmon
Sesame seeds
Strawberries
Sea salt
Spinach
Scallion
Sunflower seeds
Smoked paprika
Sweet potato
Shallot
Sundried tomatoes
Sesame oil
Sumac
Shiitake mushrooms
Sage
Sweet paprika

Sea bass

T
Turmeric
Tapioca flour
Tomato
Trout
Turkey
Thyme
Tuna
Tarragon
Turkey breast
Tilapia fillets
Tart cherries

V
Vanilla extract
Vegetable stock

W
Walnuts
Whole-wheat bread
White beans
White pepper

Z
Zucchinis

Measurement Conversion Table

CUP	OUNCES	MILLILITERS	TABLESPOONS
8 cup	64 oz.	1895 ml	128
6 cup	48 oz.	1420 ml	96
5 cup	40 oz.	1180 ml	80
4 cup	32 oz.	960 ml	64
2 cup	16 oz.	480 ml	32
1 cup	8 oz.	240 ml	16
3/4 cup	6 oz.	177 ml	12
2/3 cup	5 oz.	158 ml	11
1/2 cup	4 oz.	118 ml	8
3/8 cup	3 oz.	90 ml	6
1/3 cup	2.5 oz.	79 ml	5.5
1/4 cup	2 oz.	59 ml	4
1/8 cup	1 oz.	30 ml	3
1/16 cup	1/2 oz.	15 ml	1

Conclusion

Congratulations on finishing this book; the "Anti-Inflammatory Cookbook for Beginners" is a comprehensive guide and a useful resource for anybody seeking to enhance their health and well-being through an anti-inflammatory diet. Understanding the ideas and advantages of an anti-inflammatory diet, as well as integrating the tasty and nutritious recipes presented in this book, can help you improve your eating habits and embrace a healthy lifestyle.

You've discovered a wide range of delectable and gratifying meals in this cookbook that are specifically designed to reduce inflammation in the body. Each meal, from vivid salads and robust soups to nourishing main dishes and tempting desserts, has been meticulously prepared to not only tickle your taste buds but also nourish your body from within.

You have learned how to decrease or eliminate foods known to promote inflammation, such as processed meats, refined sugars, and trans fats, by following the principles of the anti-inflammatory diet. Instead, you've embraced various anti-inflammatory foods, such as colorful fruits and vegetables, whole grains, lean proteins, and healthy fats. These substances work together to reduce inflammation, improve your immune system, and promote overall well-being.

Furthermore, this cookbook has provided practical advice for meal planning, time management, and kitchen organization, making the anti-inflammatory diet easier to implement into your daily life than ever before. You have set yourself up for success on your quest to better health and vigor by planning and preparing balanced meals.

Remember that consistency and balance are essential as you embark on your anti-inflammatory path. Small, steady dietary changes can have a big impact on your overall health and wellness. Listen to your body, respect its requirements, and be careful of your eating choices.

With the "Anti-Inflammatory Cookbook for Beginners," you now have the information, tools, and recipes to begin a lifelong path of nourishing your body and lowering inflammation. Accept this new way of eating, taste the flavors, and rejoice in the beneficial changes in your health and well-being.

May this cookbook be your dependable companion on your anti-inflammatory journey, and may your culinary excursions be filled with brilliant flavors, plenty of energy, and a refreshed sense of vigor? Cheers to a happier, healthier you!

Recipe Index

Made in United States
Troutdale, OR
01/10/2024

16875343R00064